Quick Look Series IN VETERINARY MEDICINE

VETERINARY HISTOLOGY

Jo Ann C. Eurell, DVM, MS, PhD

Associate Professor of Morphology
College of Veterinary Medicine
University of Illinois
Urbana, Illinois

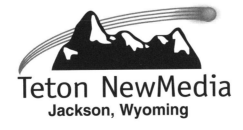

Teton NewMedia
Jackson, Wyoming

Executive Editor: Carroll C. Cann
Development Editor: Susan L. Hunsberger
Editor: Nicol Giandomenico
Art Director and Production Manager: Anita B. Sykes
Illustrations: Janet Sinn-Hanlon
Production and Layout: 5640 Design www.fiftysixforty.com
Printer: Printers Inc. Salt Lake City UT

Teton NewMedia
P.O. Box 4833
4125 South Hwy 89, Suite 1
Jackson, WY 83001
1-888-770-3165
www.veterinarywire.com

Library of Congress Cataloging-in-Publication Data

Eurell, Jo Ann Coers.
  Veterinary histology / Jo Ann C. Eurell.
    p. cm. - - (Quick look series in veterinary medicine)
  ISBN 1-893441-93-8 (alk. paper)
    1. Veterinary histology. I. Title. II. Series.

  SF757.3.E97 2003
  636.89'1018- -dc22   2003061242

PRINTED IN THE UNITED STATES OF AMERICA

ISBN # 1-893441-95-4 (bundle)

Print number 5 4 3 2 1

Table of Contents

Dedication

Through this book, I hope veterinary students will gain a better understanding of the animal body at the microscopic level. Thank you to Nicol Giandomenico, John Febiger Spahr and Carroll Cann for believing in the project. Thank you also to Janet Hanlon for creative artwork that put my vision on paper. Professors R. Hullinger, D. Van Sickle and W. Haensly deserve credit for opening my eyes to the subject and challenging me along the way. Behind every author of every book is a family who makes it possible. I would like to thank the Eurell family - Thomas for constant love and support, Joan for her enthusiasm, David for making suggestions on what to write, and Rosemarie, Adam, Lisa, Aaron, Ashley, and Victoria for being there.

Quick Look Series IN VETERINARY MEDICINE

VETERINARY HISTOLOGY

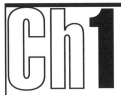

The Cell

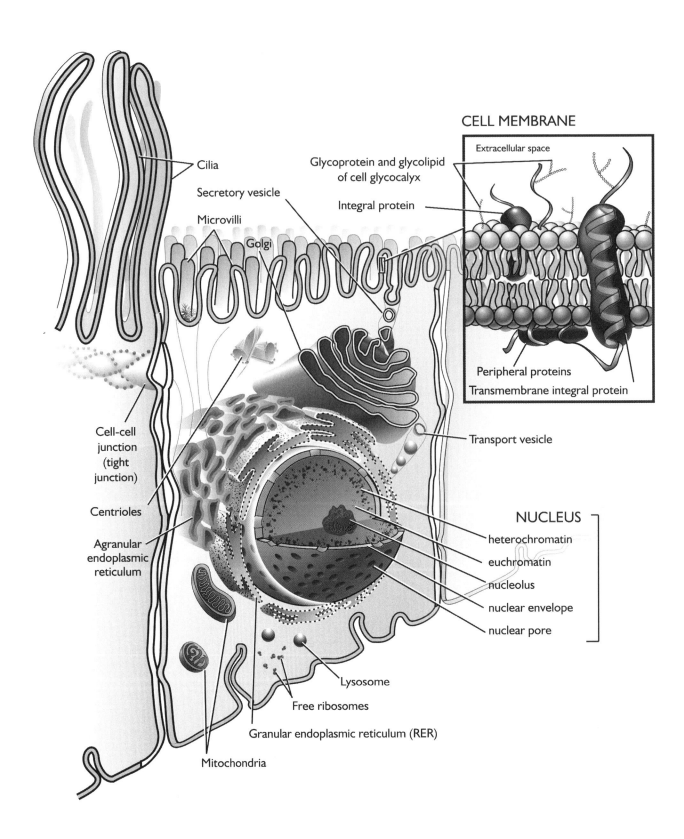

Cilia

Secretory vesicle

Microvilli

Golgi

Cell-cell
junction
(tight
junction)

Centrioles

Agranular
endoplasmic
reticulum

CELL MEMBRANE

Glycoprotein and glycolipid
of cell glycocalyx

Integral protein

Extracellular space

Peripheral proteins

Transmembrane integral protein

Transport vesicle

NUCLEUS

heterochromatin

euchromatin

nucleolus

nuclear envelope

nuclear pore

Lysosome

Free ribosomes

Granular endoplasmic reticulum (RER)

Mitochondria

Overview

- The cell is the basic structural unit of tissues.
- A lipid bilayer with embedded proteins forms the cell membrane.
- The nucleus controls cell function.
- Granular endoplasmic reticulum and associated ribosomes produce proteins.
- Agranular endoplasmic reticulum is associated with steroid production and detoxification.
- The Golgi complex packages protein for export.
- Mitochondria provide energy for the cell.
- Cell surface modifications include microvilli, cilia, flagella and stereocilia.

The cell is the basic structural unit of the tissues and organs of the body. Various cell shapes include spherical, stellate, spindle, polyhedral, squamous, cuboidal or columnar. Cell sizes range from a single micrometer to several centimeters in diameter.

Cell Membrane

Each cell in the body is bounded by a **cell membrane** (plasmalemma) which provides a barrier and controls movement of substances into and out of the cell. The cell membrane is a lipid bilayer with embedded proteins. **Integral proteins** are tightly bound within the membrane and often extend across it as transmembrane proteins. These transmembrane proteins frequently form ion channels or carrier proteins that transport molecules across the cell membrane. **Peripheral proteins,** located on the cytoplasmic surface of the cell membrane, are more loosely bound to other membrane proteins or lipids. A **glycocalyx,** comprised of carbohydrates on the outer surface of the cell membrane, functions in cell recognition, adhesion, absorption and antigenicity.

Nucleus

More than one **nucleus** can be present in a cell. Within this spherical structure, deoxyribonucleic acid (DNA) is transcribed and ribonucleic acid (RNA) is synthesized. The surrounding **nuclear envelope** is formed by two adjacent bilaminar lipid membranes with embedded proteins. Scattered **nuclear pores,** which perforate the envelope, regulate passage of substances between the cytoplasm and the nucleus. **Chromatin,** primarily comprised of DNA, is located within the nucleus. The inert form of chromatin, **heterochromatin,** stains intensely while **euchromatin,** which is actively involved in protein production, stains lightly. Nuclear chromatin condenses to form **chromosomes** during cell division. Also within the nucleus is the **nucleolus** that is the site of rRNA synthesis. The number and size of cell nucleoli are related to the amount of protein synthesis occurring within the cell.

Cytoplasm

The **cytoplasm,** which surrounds the nucleus and the organelles of the cell, varies in composition of water, protein, carbohydrates and salts. A **cytoskeleton** of microfilaments, intermediate filaments and microtubles provides structure for cell shape and movement.

Organelles and Inclusions

In the cytoplasm, **granular endoplasmic reticulum** (rough endoplasmic reticulum, rER) is comprised of membranous cisternae with attached **ribosomes**. The ribosomes, made up of ribosomal RNA, translate messenger RNA from the nucleus. As a result of the translation, specific proteins are formed within the lumen of the cisternae and are subsequently packaged for export outside the cell. Free ribosomes may also be present in the cytoplasm and function in the production of intracellular proteins. **Agranular endoplasmic reticulum** (smooth endoplasmic reticulum, sER) lacks ribosomes and is associated with glycogen synthesis, steroid production and cell detoxification.

The **Golgi complex,** a curved stack of membranes in the cytoplasm, receives protein-containing transport vesicles from the rER on the convex surface and releases secretory vesicles from the concave surface. While passing through the Golgi complex, proteins are glycosylated, phosphorylated or sulfated in preparation for export.

Mitochondria have a smooth outer membrane while the inner membrane is folded into characteristic **cristae.** Matrix granules are also present. Mitochondria produce chemical energy for the cell through the tricarboxylic acid cycle, oxidative phosphorylation and fatty acid oxidation.

Membrane-bounded structures known as **lysosomes** contain hydrolytic enzymes which help remove debris, spent organelles, and other substances from the cell. **Peroxisomes** are similar to lysosomes but contain oxidative enzymes.

Many different types of **vesicles** containing material being transported through the cell are also present in the cytoplasm. These vesicles may be coated with materials such as clathrin or coatomer. The vesicles shuttle between the cell surface, Golgi apparatus, granular endoplasmic reticulum or lysosomes depending on the transport pathway.

Other **inclusions** within the cell often include secretory granules, nutrients such as glycogen and lipid, and pigments.

Cell Surface Modifications

Depending on cell shape and function, the surface membrane may be modified to form special structures. **Microvilli** are short, finger-like projections of the cell membrane which are non-motile, but dramatically increase cell surface area for absorptive functions. **Stereocilia** are long microvilli limited to the epididymis and ear. **Cilia** and longer **flagella** contain microtubules arranged in a characteristic pattern. Nine pairs of microtubules occupy the periphery of the cilium or flagellum while one pair is found in the center. Both cilia and flagella are motile. Another cilium-like structure, the **kinocilium,** is found in the ear.

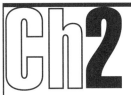

Cell Cycle

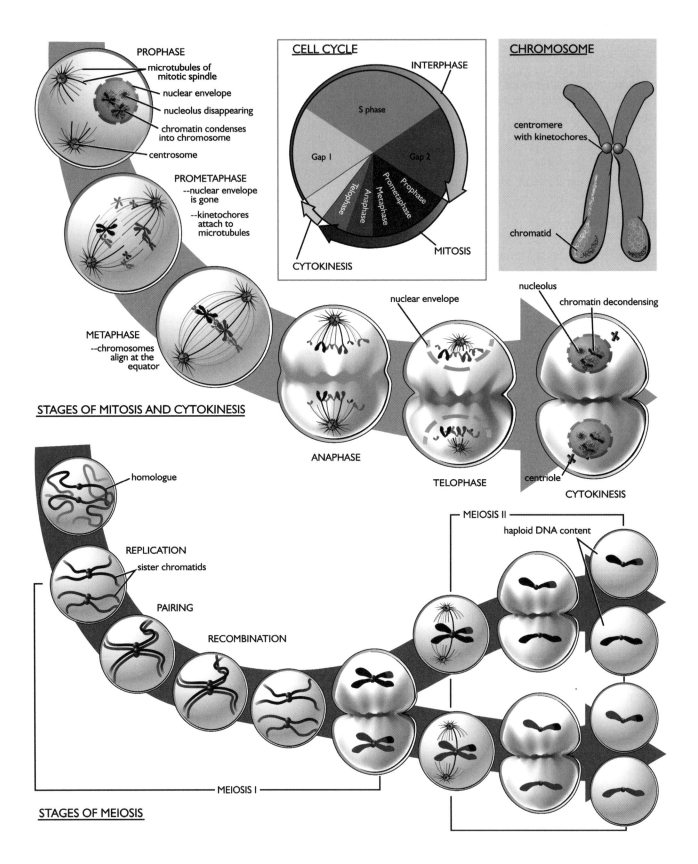

PROPHASE
- microtubules of mitotic spindle
- nuclear envelope
- nucleolus disappearing
- chromatin condenses into chromosome
- centrosome

PROMETAPHASE
- --nuclear envelope is gone
- --kinetochores attach to microtubules

METAPHASE
- --chromosomes align at the equator

STAGES OF MITOSIS AND CYTOKINESIS

CELL CYCLE

INTERPHASE

S phase

Gap 1   Gap 2

Telophase
Anaphase
Metaphase
Prometaphase
Prophase

MITOSIS

CYTOKINESIS

CHROMOSOME

centromere with kinetochores

chromatid

nuclear envelope

nucleolus

chromatin decondensing

ANAPHASE

TELOPHASE

centriole

CYTOKINESIS

homologue

REPLICATION
- sister chromatids

PAIRING

RECOMBINATION

MEIOSIS II

haploid DNA content

MEIOSIS I

STAGES OF MEIOSIS

Overview

- The cell cycle of dividing cells includes interphase, mitosis, and cytokinesis.
- During interphase, the cell undergoes growth and synthesis of DNA and RNA.
- Interphase is divided into Gap1, S and Gap 2 phases.
- Mitosis has 5 phases: prophase, prometaphase, metaphase, anaphase, and telophase.
- Cytokinesis, or division of the cell cytoplasm, results in two daughter cells.
- Reduction of chromosome numbers to half the diploid state occurs during meiosis.
- Apoptosis is programmed cell death.

The cell cycle prepares the cell for division. Most cells in the body are capable of division, but some cells, such as neurons, do not divide once cellular maturity is reached. The cycle of dividing cells includes **interphase, mitosis** and **cytokinesis.** Initiation of the cell cycle is governed by proteins known as cyclins and associated **cyclin-dependent kinases** (CDKs).

Interphase

During interphase, the cell undergoes growth, RNA synthesis, and DNA synthesis. **Gap 1** (G_1) of interphase is the time period when proteins necessary for DNA replication and enzymes are synthesized. As a result of this synthesis, the cell increases in size.

The cell continues into **S phase** during which nucleoproteins and histones are assembled into DNA. DNA is replicated into pairs of chromosomes in preparation for future cell division. The chromosomal pairs are comprised of two sister **chromatids** joined at a **centromere.**

During **Gap 2** (G_2) phase, the RNA and proteins needed for cell division are synthesized.

Mitosis

Mitosis is the segregation of chromosomes and the formation of two separate nuclei within a dividing cell.

The **prophase** portion of mitosis begins with the appearance of condensed chromosomes and the dispersion of the nucleolus. In the cytoplasm, the cytoskeleton of the cell disassembles followed by the formation of the **mitotic spindle.** Two **centrosomes,** comprised of centrioles and matrix, are the anchor points for the microtubules of the mitotic spindle apparatus.

The nuclear envelope disappears as **prometaphase** begins. Kinetochores on the centromere of each chromosome attach to the microtubules of the mitotic spindle and tension is exerted on the chromosome.

During **metaphase,** the chromosomes are aligned on the equatorial plane (metaphase plate) of the dividing cell by the paired microtubules.

Sister chromatids separate quickly during **anaphase.** The resulting individual chromatids migrate to opposite poles of the cell.

The nuclear envelopes and nucleoli of the new cells begin to reappear during **telophase.** Kinetochore microtubules disappear and chromosomes uncoil to form heterochromatin and euchromatin.

Cytokinesis

During late anaphase, a cleavage furrow forms in the plasma membrane at the site where the cell will divide. At the end of telophase, the cell undergoes **cytokinesis** resulting in two separate but identical daughter cells.

Meiosis

Meiosis is specialized cell division which results in the reduction of chromosome numbers from diploid (2n) to haploid (1n) state. The process of meiosis involves two nuclear divisions instead of one. This type of cell division occurs during the formation of ovocytes and spermatozoa. As germ cells combine at fertilization, diploid state is reestablished and genetic diversity is perpetuated by the sharing of chromosomes from two parents.

The diploid nucleus contains two similar versions of each chromosome: one maternal homologue and one paternal homologue. **Meiosis I** includes replication of the homologues which then pair. During pairing, genetic recombination may occur. The paired homologues line up at the spindle and then separate such that recombined sister chromatids migrate to opposite poles of the dividing cell.

During **meiosis II,** the two sister chromatids in each of the daughter cells separate and migrate to opposite poles. Four new haploid cells then form.

Apoptosis

Cells in the body are genetically programmed to die in response to certain accumulated injuries or aging. This programed cell death, called **apoptosis,** is governed by genes which code for enzymes called **caspases.** The caspases are induced when cytokines bind to cell receptors. The binding initiates caspase production followed by cell breakdown.

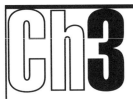

Cell Signaling

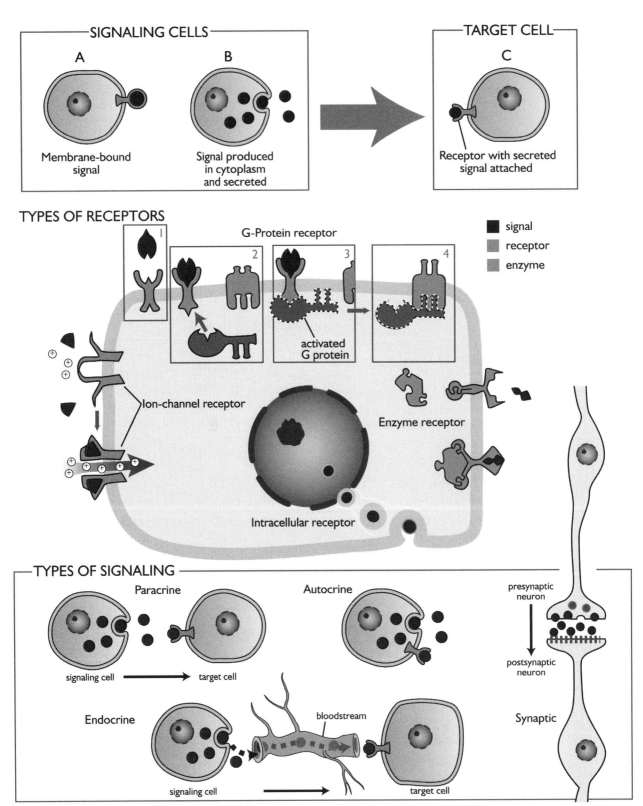

Overview

- Signals can be bound to the cell membrane or released from its cytoplasm.
- Target cells respond to signals in a specific way.
- Receptors can be linked to an ion channel, G-protein, or enzyme or they can be intracellular.
- Types of cell signaling include paracrine, endocrine, autocrine and synaptic.

Cells communicate with each other through cell signaling. Signals such as proteins, amino acids or steroids are either bound to the cell membrane of a **signaling cell** (A) or released from the cytoplasm of the signaling cell (B). The **target cell** (C) then either receives the membrane-bound signal which is still attached to the signaling cell or it receives the secreted signaling molecules. The signals attach to the target cell at specific surface proteins called **receptors.**

Each target cell is programmed to respond in a specific way to a given set of signals. When deprived of appropriate signals, the cell will undergo programmed cell death, also known as apoptosis.

Receptors

Three types of receptors, located either on the surface or within target cells, receive signals from other cells. **Ion-channel-linked receptors** receive a signal and then change configuration to allow the passage of ions through a channel in the cell membrane. When a **G-protein-linked receptor** is activated by a signal molecule, the G-protein mediates the activity of another membrane-bound target protein (an enzyme or an ion channel). Upon signaling, **enzyme-linked receptors** either function directly as enzymes or are linked with enzymes which are activated to catalyze a specific chemical reaction within the cell.

The three classes of surface receptors receive signals and relay the signals to the cell nucleus through an elaborate set of **intracellular signaling proteins (ISPs).** At the nucleus, the received signals alter the expression of certain genes which govern the behavior of the cell.

Intracellular receptors are located within the cell rather than on the surface of the cell membrane. Small signaling molecules (steroid hormones, thyroid hormone, vitamin D) diffuse across the cell membrane and bind to receptors located inside the cell in either the nucleus or the cytoplasm. The activated intracellular receptors then regulate the transcription of specific genes.

Gap Junctions and Signaling

Gap junctions are specialized junctions between the plasma membranes of neighboring cells (see Epithelium). These intercellular channels allow exchange of small molecules between cells. The molecular exchange helps coordinate behaviors of similar groups of cells.

Signaling Types

In **paracrine signaling,** a signaling cell produces molecules which affect neighboring target cells. The signaling molecules diffuse a short distance from the producing cell. **Endocrine signaling** involves production of a signal, or hormone, which moves from the signaling cell to a target cell via the bloodstream. The target cell may be some distance from where the signal was initially produced. **Autocrine signaling** takes place in cells which produce a signal that binds back to the producing cell. Autocrine signaling works best when a group of cells carry out the signaling simultaneously. Therefore, autocrine signaling is thought to help clusters of developing cells respond whereas a single cell could not. Eicosanoids are autocrine signals which act in mature tissues. **Synaptic signaling** involves the activity of neurons which conduct electrical impulses resulting in the release of neurotransmitter signals which travel across the synaptic gap between cells.

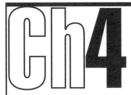
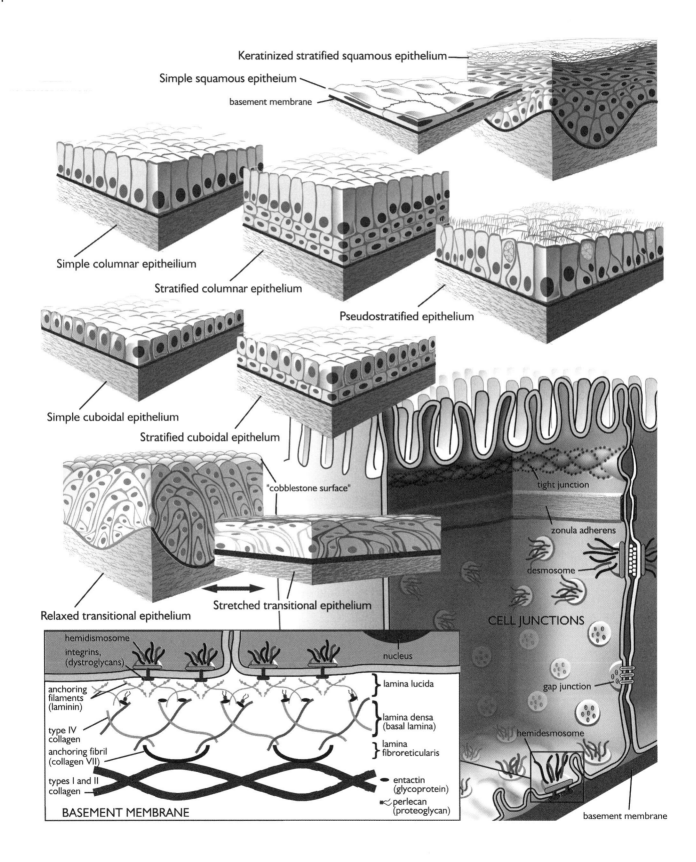

Keratinized stratified squamous epithelium

Simple squamous epitheium

basement membrane

Simple columnar epitheilium

Stratified columnar epithelium

Pseudostratified epithelium

Simple cuboidal epithelium

Stratified cuboidal epithelum

"cobblestone surface"

tight junction

zonula adherens

desmosome

Relaxed transitional epithelium

Stretched transitional epithelium

CELL JUNCTIONS

gap junction

hemidismosome

integrins, (dystroglycans)

nucleus

lamina lucida

anchoring filaments (laminin)

lamina densa (basal lamina)

type IV collagen

anchoring fibril (collagen VII)

lamina fibroreticularis

types I and II collagen

entactin (glycoprotein)

perlecan (proteoglycan)

hemidesmosome

BASEMENT MEMBRANE

basement membrane

Overview

- Epithelium is comprised of avascular sheets of cells with little intercellular substance.
- Simple epithelia have a single layer of cells while stratified epithelia are multilayered.
- Epithelia are further classified by the shape of the cells in the surface layer: squamous cells are flattened, cuboidal cells are cube-shaped, and columnar cells are taller than they are wide.
- In pseudostratified epithelium, all cells contact the basement membrane but many cells do not reach the surface of the epithelium.
- The appearance of transitional epithelium changes as it relaxes or stretches.
- The basement membrane is comprised of the lamina lucida, lamina densa and lamina fibroreticularis.
- Cell junctions include the tight junction, zonula adherens, desmosome, hemidesmosome and gap

The tissues of the body can each be classified as one of four basic tissues: **epithelium, connective tissue, muscle or nervous tissue.**

An **epithelium** is a sheet of cells which lines a lumen of an organ or covers an organ surface. The tissue is avascular, highly cellular, and has little intercellular substance. Epithelia protect underlying structures and function in absorption, secretion, surface transport, and sensory reception. Each epithelium is classified by the number of cellular layers and the shape of cells in the surface layer.

Simple Epithelium

A simple epithelium consists of a single layer of cells. The cells of **simple squamous epithelium** are flat. The nuclear region of the squamous epithelial cell protrudes while surrounding cytoplasmic areas of the cell are thin. Simple squamous epithelium is termed **mesothelium** when lining body cavities and **endothelium** when lining cardiovascular structures. **Simple cuboidal epithelial cells** are cube-shaped in contrast to **simple columnar epithelial** cells which are tall and narrow. Simple cuboidal epithelium lines excretory ducts while simple columnar epithelium is associated with absorptive functions in the intestine and other organs.

Stratified Epithelium

A stratified epithelium has multiple cell layers. Only the basal layer of cells contacts the underlying basement membrane. Epithelium in this category is further classified by the shape of the cells in the surface layer of the tissue. **Stratified squamous epithelium** varies both in number of cell layers and in thickness depending on the location in the body. When cells in the surface layers of stratified squamous epithelium lack nuclei and have increased keratin in their cytoplasm, the epithelium is described as **keratinized**. Skin is a typical example of keratinized, stratified squamous epithelium. **Stratified cuboidal epithelium** is usually limited to two cell layers and is typically found in large excretory ducts. The surface layer of this epithelium is made up of cuboidal cells. Stratified columnar epithelium has columnar cells in the surface layer. Rarely found in the body, this epithelium is confined to large ducts and some regions of the urethra.

Pseudostratifed Epithelium

All cells in **pseudostratified epithelium** contact the underlying basement membrane, but many of the cells do not reach to the surface of the epithelium. Nuclei of the epithelial cells are at different levels within the epithelium. Most pseudostratified epithelium is also ciliated. This epithelium is found in the respiratory system.

Transitional Epithelium

Transitional epithelium is also considered pseudostratified. This epithelium is found in urinary system organs which expand and contract. In the stretched condition, transitional epithelium flattens but in the relaxed state, the epithelial cells appear to be stacked and protrude into the lumen. The domed appearance of the surface epithelial cells is characteristic of transitional epithelium.

Basement Membrane

Epithelial cells attach to a **basement membrane** which anchors the epithelium to underlying structures and plays an important role in epithelial regeneration after injury. The basement membrane appears as a dense, acellular region when viewed with the light microscope, but it resolves into three layers with electron microscopy. The **lamina lucida** (lamina rara) is an unstained area between the basal cell membrane of the epithelial cells and the underlying lamina densa. Laminin anchoring filaments are located in the lamina lucida. The **lamina densa** (basal lamina) consists of a dense, heavily-stained network of type IV collagen linked to laminin by proteoglycans and glycoproteins. The lamina densa contacts the underlying **lamina fibroreticularis** which is comprised of anchoring fibrils and interwoven collagen fibers extending from the underlying connective tissue.

Cell Junctions

Epithelial cells are joined together by a variety of cell junctions. The lateral cell membranes near the surface of the epithelium fuse to form the encircling **tight junction** (zona occludens). Intercellular space is obliterated by the tight junction and passage of material between cells is not allowed. The **zonula adherens** also encircles the cell but a space of 15-20 nm is present between the cell membranes. Cadherin molecules span the intercellular space and bind to actin filaments within the adjacent cells thus establishing a secure cell junction. Epithelial cells are also joined by randomly distributed patch junctions called **desmosomes** (macula adherens), comprised of cadherins linked to intermediate filaments. Along the basal border of epithelium, **hemidesmosomes** (integrins linked to intermediate filaments) and **adhesion placques** (integrins linked to actin microfilaments) anchor the cells to the basement membrane. The **gap junction** (nexus or communicating junction) is scattered on the lateral surface of many epithelial cells. Six transmembrane proteins called connexons surround a central pore through which ions and small molecules move from one cell to another.

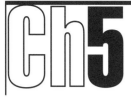

Glands

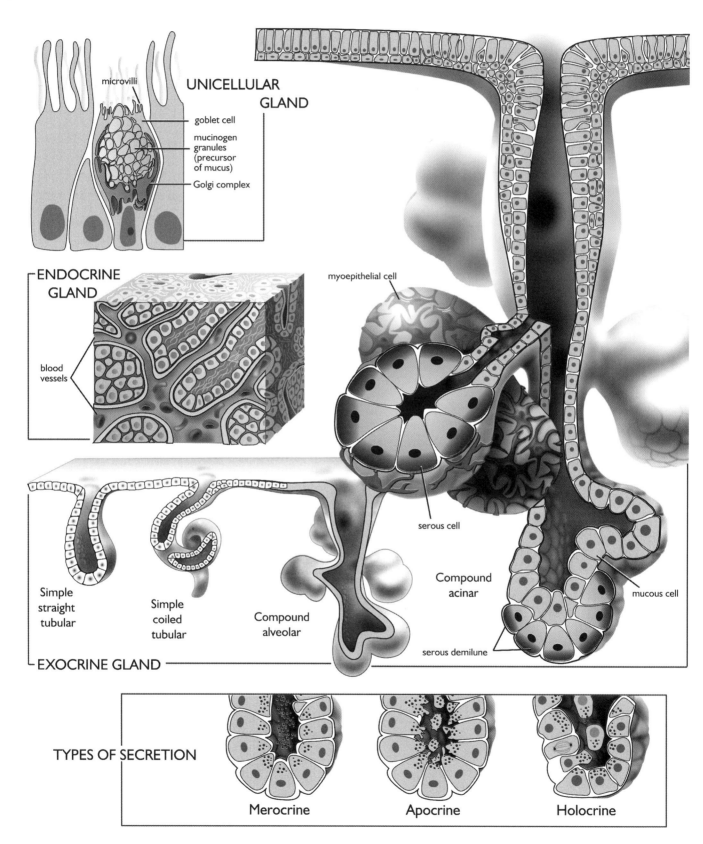

UNICELLULAR GLAND

microvilli

goblet cell

mucinogen granules (precursor of mucus)

Golgi complex

ENDOCRINE GLAND

blood vessels

myoepithelial cell

serous cell

Compound acinar

mucous cell

serous demilune

Simple straight tubular

Simple coiled tubular

Compound alveolar

EXOCRINE GLAND

TYPES OF SECRETION

Merocrine

Apocrine

Holocrine

Overview

- Unicellular glands are single cells while multicellular glands contain multiple cells and include large organs.
- Endocrine glands lack ducts and secrete directly into circulating blood while exocrine glands have a secretory duct system which transports the product from the gland.
- Simple glands have an unbranched duct system while the duct system of compound glands is branched.
- Secretory units can be classified as tubular, acinar or alveolar based on shape.
- The modes of glandular secretion are merocrine, apocrine or holocrine.
- Secretory products of certain glands are described as serous, mucous or mixed.

Classification of Glands

Unicellular glands are single cells that secrete product directly from the cell. The product may affect adjacent cells (paracrine signaling) or may be transported some distance away from the secretory cell. An example of a unicellular gland is the **goblet cell** which produces mucus. Goblet cells are scattered between other epithelial cells in many locations throughout the body.

Multicellular glands contain multiple secretory cells. The functional cells of the gland are known as **parenchyma** while the supporting connective tissue is **stroma.** Multicellular glands range from small sweat glands to large organs such as the pancreas.

Endocrine vs. Exocrine Glands

Endocrine glands secrete their product directly into the circulating blood which delivers the product to target cells. The duct system is lacking in endocrine glands but is an important feature of **exocrine glands.** The thyroid is an endocrine gland while salivary glands are exocrine.

Exocrine Ducts

The duct system of exocrine glands is lined by epithelium which ranges in height from low simple cuboidal epithelium near the secretory units to stratified columnar epithelium in larger ducts.

Duct structure is further described as either **simple** or **compound.** A simple gland has an unbranched duct system while the duct system of a compound gland branches repeatedly.

Secretory Units

Secretory units of exocrine glands are classified as **tubular, acinar or alveolar.** Epithelium of a **tubule** is arranged as a cylinder with a narrow central lumen. By comparison, epithelium of an **acinus** forms a sac-like structure with a small lumen while an **alveolus** has a large lumen. The epithelial cells lining the secretory units are polarized to secrete their product into the lumen.

Myoepithelial cells surround the secretory epithelium of some glands. These cells are located between the basal membrane of the epithelial cells and the adjacent basement membrane complex. Myoepithelial cells contract, thereby helping to expel the secretory product from the epithelial cells.

Mode of Secretion

During secretion, a varying amount of the glandular epithelial cell is lost. In **merocrine** secretion, the cell product is secreted while the epithelial cells remain intact. A portion of the epithelial cell is lost with the product of apocrine glands while the entire secretory cell is shed in holocrine secretion.

Serous vs. Mucous Secretion

The secretory product of certain glands can be characterized as either **serous** or **mucous.**

Serous secretion is watery in consistency and rich in protein. Glands which produce serous substances typically have a basophilic cytoplasm due to a high concentration of granular endoplasmic reticulum related to the secretory process. The nucleus of the secretory cell is located in the basal cytoplasm and is spherical.

In contrast, **mucus,** the product of mucous glands, is viscous and rich in carbohydrates. Mucous cells have a very light staining cytoplasm due to the accumulation of the mucus prior to secretion. In comparison to the serous cell, the nucleus is also basally located in the mucous cell but it is flattened instead of spherical.

Some glands have both serous and mucous cells in their secretory units. These glands are considered **mixed** and produce a seromucous secretion. The serous and mucous cells can be intermixed within the secretory epithelium or the secretory cells can be predominately mucous with crescent-shaped aggregate of serous cells known as a **serous demilune.** Serous secretions from the demilunes reach the lumen of the adenomere via intercellular canaliculi which pass between the mucous cells.

In addition to serous and mucous products, glands produce a wide variety of other products including hormones, enzymes, etc. which will be discussed with the specific organ.

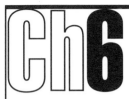

Connective Tissue

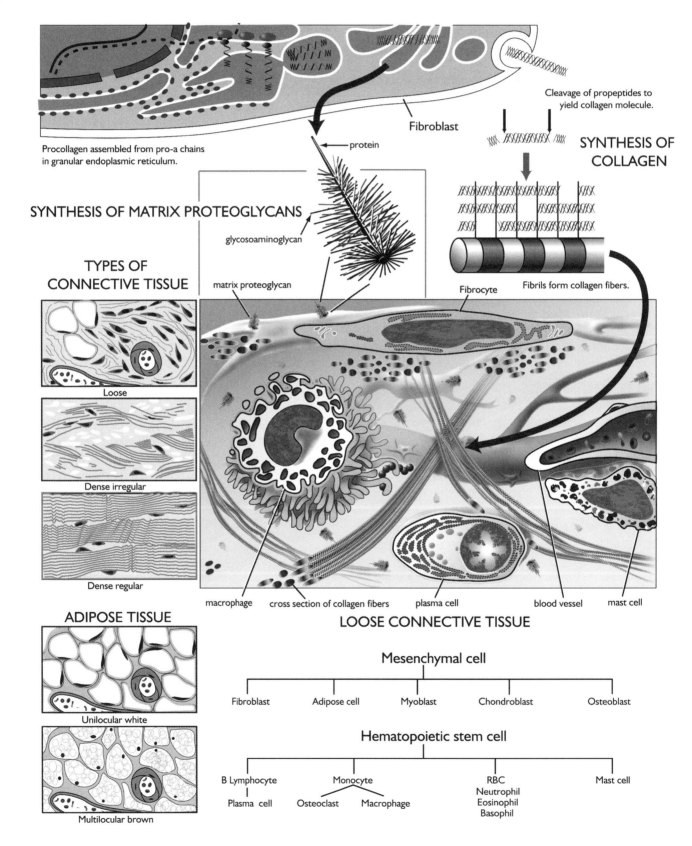

Procollagen assembled from pro-a chains in granular endoplasmic reticulum.

Fibroblast

protein

Cleavage of propeptides to yield collagen molecule.

SYNTHESIS OF COLLAGEN

SYNTHESIS OF MATRIX PROTEOGLYCANS

glycosoaminoglycan

matrix proteoglycan

TYPES OF CONNECTIVE TISSUE

Loose

Dense irregular

Dense regular

Fibrocyte

Fibrils form collagen fibers.

macrophage   cross section of collagen fibers   plasma cell   blood vessel   mast cell

LOOSE CONNECTIVE TISSUE

ADIPOSE TISSUE

Unilocular white

Multilocular brown

Mesenchymal cell

Fibroblast   Adipose cell   Myoblast   Chondroblast   Osteoblast

Hematopoietic stem cell

B Lymphocyte   Monocyte   RBC   Mast cell
                              Neutrophil
Plasma cell   Osteoclast   Macrophage   Eosinophil
                              Basophil

Overview

- Connective tissue provides support and structural framework for the body.
- Cells include fibroblasts, fibrocytes, mesenchymal cells, mast cells, plasma cells, macrophages, adipose cells, pigment cells, reticular cells and pericytes.
- Fibers of connective tissue proper are collagen, reticular fibers, elastic fibers and fibrous adhesive proteins.
- Ground substance which fills in between the fibers includes glycosaminoglycans and proteoglycans.
- Connective tissue is classified as loose, dense irregular and dense regular connective tissue.
- White fat and brown fat are two types of adipose tissue.

Connective tissue provides support and structure for the body and it participates in heat regulation, defense and repair processes. Fibers and ground substance predominate over cells in this tissue.

Cells of Connective Tissue Proper

The spindle-shaped **fibroblast** produces the fibers and ground substance of connective tissue proper. In a less active state, the cell is referred to as a **fibrocyte.**

The **mesenchymal cell,** an undifferentiated precursor cell, has the potential to develop into one of several different cells. The mesenchymal cell is smaller than the fibroblast and has a prominent euchromatic nucleus.

Mast cells are unique connective tissue cells which produce and store granules of heparin, histamine and other factors. At the light microscopic level, the granules often obscure the nucleus and are distinctly metachromatic when stained with toluidine blue.

Plasma cells migrate freely in connective tissue. These cells represent highly-differentiated B lymphocytes which produce immunoglobulins. The plasma cell is spherical with an eccentric heterochromatic nucleus and well-developed granular reticulum in the cytoplasm.

Macrophages can be fixed or migratory in connective tissue. This cell develops from the monocyte and has an indented nucleus, lysosomes, and vacuoles in the cytoplasm. Macrophages are phagocytic and synthesize many diverse factors.

Adipose cells contain large amounts of lipid in their cytoplasm. Unilocular adipose cells have one large lipid droplet and the nucleus is compressed to the periphery of the cell. In contrast, multilocular adipose cells contain several smaller lipid droplets.

Other connective tissue cells include **pigment cells** which contain various pigments such as melanin; **reticular cells** which form the supportive framework in lymphoid organs and bone marrow; and **pericytes** which surround blood vessels and regulate their diameter.

Fibers of Connective Tissue Proper

The predominate fiber of connective tissue matrix is **collagen.**

Fibril-forming collagen includes types I, II, III, V and XI. Type I collagen is predominate in connective tissue proper. Collagen molecules are assembled into collagen fibrils outside the fibroblast where they are produced. Alignment of the mol-ecules within the fibril yields characteristic ultrastructural striations in some collagens. Fibrils are further assembled into collagen fibers. Collagen stains pink with standard hematoxylin and eosin stain.

Network-forming collagen forms a flexible framework for the basal lamina of epithelia. This class of collagens includes types IV and VII.

Fibril-associated collagen may mediate interaction between collagen fibrils and other matrix components. This group of collagens includes types IX and XII.

Reticular fibers are small, type III collagen fibers which are produced by fibroblasts and certain reticular cells. These fibers are coated with proteoglycans and glycoproteins which attract silver stains.

Elastic fibers are composed of elastin, which allows the fiber to stretch and then return to the original configuration when released. With hematoxylin and eosin stain, elastic fibers stain orange and are refractile under light microscopy.

Fibronectin and laminin are two of several non-collagenous **fibrous adhesive proteins.** Fibronectin mediates connection between the cytoskeleton and the extracellular matrix. Laminin is a component of the lamina lucida of the basement membrane complex.

Ground Substance of Connective Tissue Proper

Glycosaminoglycans (GAGs) and proteoglycans fill the space between fibers and cells in the matrix of connective tissue proper. Major GAGs include hyaluronic acid, chondroitin sulfates, dermatan sulfate and keratan sulfate. Proteoglycans are formed by linking GAGs to a protein core.

Classification of Connective Tissue Proper

The fibers and ground substance of **loose connective tissue,** also called areolar connective tissue, are randomly arranged with considerable space in the network. Loose connective tissue is widely distributed throughout the body. **Dense irregular connective tissue** also has an irregular fiber arrangement, but less open space within the network. An example of dense irregular connective tissue is connective tissue capsules of major organs. The fibers of **dense regular connective tissue** are oriented in one direction and are tightly packed. Dense regular connective tissue is typical of tendons and ligaments.

Adipose Tissue

White adipose tissue consists of aggregates of unilocular adipose cells. This tissue is white in color when viewed grossly.

Brown adipose tissue is found in the neonate and hibernating species. The fat is brown in color and is composed of multilocular cells. Brown fat is rich in mitochondria and provides energy for thermoregulation.

Cartilage

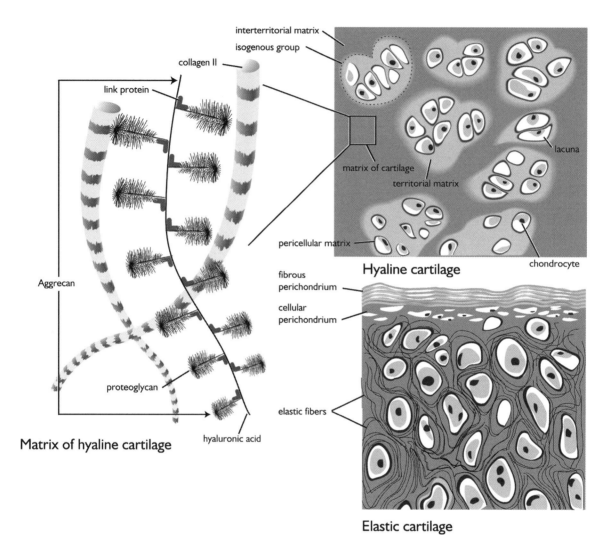

interterritorial matrix

isogenous group

collagen II

link protein

pericellular matrix

matrix of cartilage

territorial matrix

lacuna

chondrocyte

Aggrecan

proteoglycan

hyaluronic acid

Matrix of hyaline cartilage

Hyaline cartilage

fibrous perichondrium

cellular perichondrium

elastic fibers

Elastic cartilage

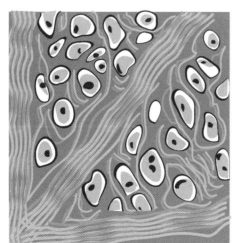

Fibrocartilage in meniscus (herringbone pattern)

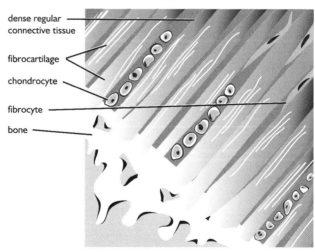

dense regular connective tissue

fibrocartilage

chondrocyte

fibrocyte

bone

Fibrocartilage at tendon insertion (unidirectional pattern)

Overview

- The cells of cartilage are chondroblasts, chondrocytes and chondroclasts.
- Chondroblasts and chondrocytes are located in lacunae.
- Type II collagen predominates in hyaline cartilage.
- Elastic fibers are present in elastic cartilage
- Type I collagen predominates in fibrocartilage.
- Perichondrium surrounds cartilage bounded by other tissues; it is absent from the articular surface.
- Cartilage is avascular.

Cartilage is a unique, semi-rigid tissue which provides supporting structure for organs such as the trachea or the ear. The tissue also forms menisci in synovial joints and creates a gliding surface on the ends of long bones. In the developing body, cartilage forms the precursor model for certain bones.

Cartilage is avascular and derives its nutrients by diffusion from surrounding tissues.

Cartilage Cells

The **chondroblast** produces matrix in growing cartilage. Chondroblasts are rich in granular endoplasmic reticulum and have a prominent Golgi complex. They are closely spaced in the tissue matrix.

Chondrocytes renew the matrix of mature cartilage. They are spherical cells with fewer organelles than the chondroblast. Chondrocytes are more widely separated in the tissue when compared to chondroblasts.

Both chondroblasts and chondrocytes reside in spaces in the semi-rigid tissue matrix called **lacunae.** When the tissue is processed for light microscopy, the cells and matrix shrink at different rates and the surrounding lacunar space becomes visible as a halo around the cell.

Chondroclasts are multi-nucleated cells which resorb cartilage. The are located adjacent to cartilage in the growth plate and may be the same cell as the osteoclast.

Cartilage Matrix

The matrix of cartilage includes fibers and ground substance.

Collagens form the fiber network of cartilage matrix. Type II collagen predominates in hyaline cartilage while type I collagen is the dominant collagen in fibrocartilage. Type VI collagen is located in the pericellular region surrounding chondrocytes while type X collagen is found in cartilage matrix which calcifies. Collagens IX, XI, XII and XIV have also been reported in cartilage matrix.

Ground substance of cartilage is comprised of large aggrecans which bind fluid and impart resiliency to the tissue. Major **glycosaminoglycans** of cartilage include chondroitin-4-sulfate, chondroitin-6-sulfate, and keratan sulfate which bind to a protein core to form a **proteoglycan.** Multiple proteoglycans are bound to hyaluronic acid by a link protein, forming the large **aggrecan.** Gel-like aggrecans occupy the space between matrix fibers.

Non-collagenous proteins include decorin, chondronectin and anchorin CII. Decorin regulates the diameter of collagen fibers during their formation while chondronectin and anchorin-CII mediate adhesion of chondrocytes to the matrix.

Types of Cartilage

Cartilage is classified based on the predominate type of fibers in the matrix.

Hyaline cartilage matrix has fine, type II collagen fibers in the matrix. These fibers are of similar refractive index to the surrounding ground substance and are not distinctly visible in the amorphous matrix.

The staining differences in the matrix of hyaline cartilage are due to variations in proteoglycan content. The **pericellular matrix** immediately surrounds the chondrocyte, forming the wall of the lacuna. This matrix region contains proteoglycans but lacks collagen. Dark-staining **territorial matrix,** comprised of proteoglycans and fine collagen fibers, is located outside the pericellular matrix region. **Interterritorial matrix** lies outside the territorial matrix and occupies the remaining matrix space. This area of matrix has larger collagen fibers with aggrecans.

The cells of hyaline cartilage are scattered in the matrix or clustered in small groups of 2 to 6 cells. These cell groups are thought to arise from the same parent cell and are called **isogenous groups** or cell nests. Chondrocytes within an isogenous groups share the same territorial matrix. Hyaline cartilage is found in the tracheal rings and articular cartilage.

The matrix of **elastic cartilage** is comprised of type II collagen and a prominent network of elastic fibers. Chondrocytes in elastic cartilage are larger than in hyaline cartilage and are scattered in less matrix. Elastic cartilage is found in the epiglottis and the pinna of the ear.

Fibrocartilage has prominent, type I collagen fibers which are arranged in either an interwoven, herringbone pattern or a unidirectional fashion. The chondrocytes are located in lacunae between the collagen fibers. Fibrocartilage is found in the intervertebral disc, joint menisci and insertions of tendons or ligaments.

Connective Tissue Associated with Cartilage

When hyaline or elastic cartilage is located adjacent to other tissues, a layer of dense connective tissue proper, known as **perichondrium,** surrounds the cartilage. The inner layer of perichondrium supplies progenitor cells to growing cartilage. The outer layer of perichondrium is dense connective tissue which provides support for the underlying cartilage. Perichondrium is not present on the gliding surface of articular cartilage or surrounding fibrocartilage.

Cartilage Growth

Cartilage can increase in size by either interstitial or appositional growth. **Interstitial growth** results from cell division and matrix formation within the cartilage model while **appositional growth** occurs on the perimeter of the model through the activity of perichondrial cells.

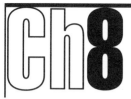

Bone

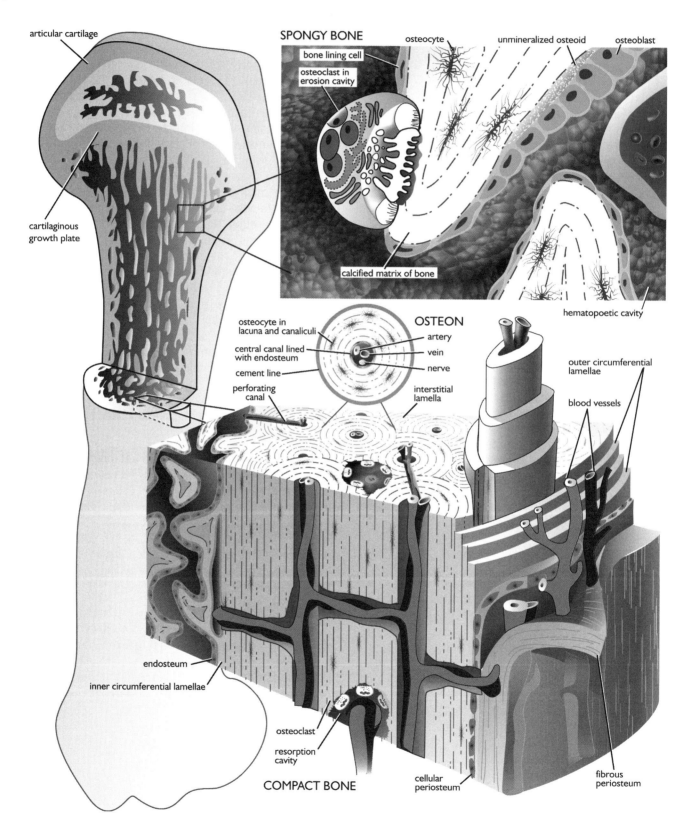

articular cartilage

cartilaginous growth plate

SPONGY BONE

bone lining cell

osteoclast in erosion cavity

osteocyte

unmineralized osteoid

osteoblast

calcified matrix of bone

hematopoetic cavity

osteocyte in lacuna and canaliculi

central canal lined with endosteum

cement line

perforating canal

OSTEON

artery

vein

nerve

interstitial lamella

outer circumferential lamellae

blood vessels

endosteum

inner circumferential lamellae

osteoclast

resorption cavity

COMPACT BONE

cellular periosteum

fibrous periosteum

Overview

- The cells of bone are the osteoblast, osteocyte and osteoclast.
- Osteocytes are located in lacunae with their cell processes extending into canaliculi.
- Osteoblasts form new bone, osteocytes maintain bone matrix, and osteoclasts resorb bone.
- The organic matrix of bone is predominately type I collagen with minimal proteoglycans and other proteins.
- Calcium salts, such as hydroxyapatite, mineralize the bone matrix.
- Compact bone is organized into cylindrical osteons.
- Interstitial lamellae occupy the spaces between osteons while circumferential lamellae cover the surfaces of compact bone.
- Spongy bone is comprised of lamellar trabeculae which lack osteons.
- Periosteum covers the outer surface of compact bone. Endosteum covers the trabeculae of spongy bone and extends into the perforating and central canals of compact bone.

Bone is a rigid tissue which, along with cartilage, forms the skeleton. In addition to functioning as a supporting structure, the bones of the skeleton protect underlying organs, provide sites for muscle and ligament attachment and serve as a reservoir for calcium.

Bone Cells

The **osteoblast** forms the matrix of bone and plays a role in matrix mineralization. Osteoblasts have single nuclei, are cuboidal to columnar in shape, and are located on bone surfaces. They are derived from mesenchymal cells. The **bone lining cell** is a squamous cell which is also found on the surfaces of adult bone and is thought to be a resting osteoblast.

As bone is formed, about 10 per cent of osteoblasts are completely surrounded by bone matrix and become **osteocytes.** These cells maintain the surrounding bone matrix and are capable of becoming osteoblasts if needed. Osteocytes are located in lacunae within the bone matrix. Multiple cell processes extend from the cell body of the osteocyte into channels in the matrix called canaliculi. Through the canaliculi, the processes of one osteocyte can contact the processes of another adjacent osteocyte.

The large, multi-nucleated **osteoclast** is responsible for bone resorption. The osteoclast occupies an **erosion cavity** (Howship's lacuna) on the surface of bone or tunnels through compact bone as the leading cell of bone remodeling units. Acidic secretions are produced by the osteoclast along its **ruffled border** which sweeps over the surface where resorption is occurring. The secretions are contained by a **clear zone,** devoid of cytoplasmic organelles, which surrounds the ruffled boarder. Two to fifty nuclei and various organelles are located in the **basal zone** of the osteoclast. A **zone of vesicles** which contain enzymes associated with resorption is located between the ruffled border and the basal zone. Osteoclasts are derived from the monocyte cell line.

Bone Matrix

Type I collagen predominates in the matrix of bone. Collagen types III, V and X are also present.

Non-collagenous proteins including alkaline phosphatase, osteonectin, gamma-carboxyglutamic acid containing proteins, osteopontin and a small amount of proteoglycans are also present.

Inorganic salts which range from calcium and phosphate ions to more complex hydroxyapatite form the mineral component of bone. The calcium salts are located in the holes and pores of the matrix collagen fibers. Due to this calcification, the matrix of bone is poorly permeable to most nutrients which must subsequently reach bone cells by flowing through the lacunar-canalicular system.

Types of Bone

Compact bone forms the cylinder surrounding the hematopoietic cavity of long bones. The tissue is organized into small cylindrical units called **osteons** (Haversian systems). Each osteon is formed by concentric lamellae or rings of matrix which surround a **central canal**. Osteocytes are located within lacunae between the lamellae. The canalicular system extends throughout the lamellae. A cement line bounds the outer margin of the osteon. Blood vessels and nerves are located in the central canal. Central canals of compact bone osteons connect to the surface of bone via **perforating canals** (Volkmann's canal) which run at right angles to the central canals.

Interstitial lamellae fill the space between osteons while **circumferential lamellae** cover the outer and inner surface of compact bone.

Spongy bone or cancellous bone is comprised of bony **trabeculae** surrounded by hematopoietic space containing bone marrow or adipose tissue. The trabeculae are avascular structures of lamellar bone. No osteons are present within trabeculae. Osteocytes of spongy bone are located in a lacunar-canalicular system similar to compact bone. Osteoblasts and osteoclasts of spongy bone are present on the surface of the trabeculae.

Connective Tissue of Bone

The outer surface of compact bone is covered by dense connective tissue called **periosteum.** The outer layer of the periosteum is dense irregular connective tissue and is referred to as the **fibrous layer.** The inner **cellular layer** adjacent to the underlying bone is made up of one or more layers of osteoblasts. Cells in this layer proliferate when the periosteum is activated during growth or injury.

Spongy bone is covered by a cellular layer known as **endosteum.** In resting bone, the bone lining cell predominates in the endosteum. Osteoblasts and osteoclasts are the primary cells of endosteum covering forming or resorbing bone surfaces. Endosteum extends from the surface of spongy bone within the marrow cavity into perforating and central canals of compact bone.

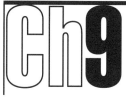

Muscle

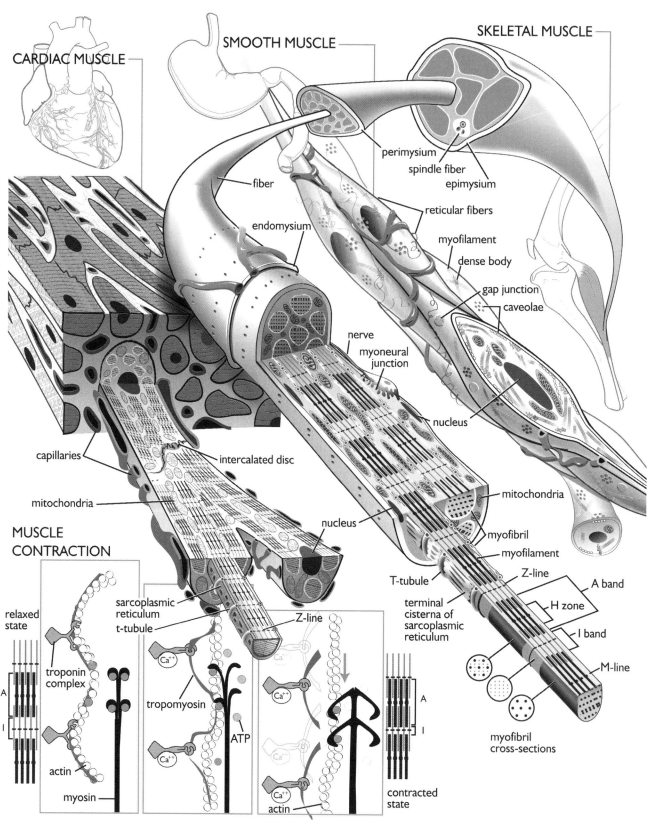

CARDIAC MUSCLE

SMOOTH MUSCLE

SKELETAL MUSCLE

perimysium
spindle fiber
epimysium
reticular fibers
myofilament
dense body
gap junction
caveolae

fiber

endomysium

nerve
myoneural
junction

nucleus

mitochondria

myofibril

myofilament

capillaries

intercalated disc

mitochondria

nucleus

MUSCLE
CONTRACTION

sarcoplasmic
reticulum
t-tubule

Z-line

T-tubule

terminal
cisterna of
sarcoplasmic
reticulum

Z-line
A band
H zone
I band
M-line

relaxed
state

troponin
complex

A

I

tropomyosin

ATP

Ca⁺⁺

Ca⁺⁺

Ca⁺⁺

Ca⁺⁺

Ca⁺⁺

A

I

myofibril
cross-sections

actin

myosin

actin

contracted
state

Overview

- Muscle fibers are the cells of muscle.
- Smooth muscle fibers are non-striated, spindle-shaped cells with a single, central nucleus.
- Skeletal muscle fibers are striated with multiple, peripherally located nuclei.
- Cardiac muscle fibers are striated with a single, centrally-located nucleus and intercalated discs.

Movement in the body is accomplished by specialized cells called muscle fibers. In addition to forming named muscles which participate in locomotion, muscle also contracts and facilitates the expression of glands and the movement of blood and gastrointestinal contents in the body. To power contraction, individual muscle cells transform chemical energy into mechanical energy by splitting ATP.

Histologic Terminology

Cells of muscle are referred to as **muscle fibers.** Within the cytoplasm, known as **sarcoplasm** in muscle, are **myofibrils** which are aggregates of **myofilaments.** Myofilaments are comprised of contractile proteins such as actin and myosin. The surrounding cell membrane is the **sarcolemma.**

Connective tissue proper which immediately surrounds a muscle fiber is **endomysium** while **perimysium** surrounds a bundle of fibers within a muscle. **Epimysium** is dense irregular connective tissue which surrounds the entire muscle.

Smooth Muscle

Smooth muscle fibers are elongated, spindle-shaped cells with a centrally located nucleus. The cells lack striations as seen in skeletal and cardiac muscle. Fine reticular fibers surround smooth muscle cells instead of a true endomysium.

With electron microscopy, the nucleus, Golgi apparatus and granular endoplasmic reticulum occupy the center of the cell while the periphery is filled with myofilaments which anchor into **dense bodies.** The sarcolemma has numerous **caveolae** and vesicles for calcium transport plus gap junctions for intercellular communication.

Smooth muscle contracts involuntarily and is capable of slow and sustained contractions.

Skeletal Muscle

With the light microscope, alternating light and dark striations are visible in skeletal muscle fibers. The light-staining band is known as the **I band** while the dark-staining band is the **A band.** The striations result from the organized arrangement of myofilaments within myofibrils. The myofibrils fill the center of the skeletal muscle fiber and are held in alignment by desmin and vimentin filaments. Multiple nuclei are displaced to the periphery of the cell. In cross sections of skeletal muscle, individual myofibrils can be seen as dots within the sarcoplasm.

With electron microscopy, the arrangement of individual myofilaments can be further observed. The A band is predominately **thick filaments** of myosin with overlapping **thin filaments** made up of actin, tropomyosin and troponin. The I band is comprised of thin filaments which are interconnected at the **Z line** located in the center of the band. A **sarcomere** extends from one Z line to the next and represents a unit of skeletal muscle contraction.

As muscle contracts, thin filaments at one end of the sarcomere slide over thick filaments toward thin filaments at the other end of the sarcomere. A light-staining region in the center of the A band, known as the **H zone,** represents an area devoid of actin filaments. Myosin myofilaments are linked together in the center of the H zone by proteins which form the **M line.**

The sarcolemma of skeletal muscle invaginates as **T tubules** (transverse tubules) which extend into the sarcoplasm. T tubules transmit electrical impulses from the surface of the cell into the interior.

Skeletal muscle fibers have extensive agranular endoplasmic reticulum, specifically known as **sarcoplasmic reticulum.** The reticulum is arranged as a network around myofibrils and forms large **terminal cisternae** at the junction of the A and I bands. A T tubule is located between two adjacent cisternae and the three structures collectively for a triad.

Skeletal muscle can contract voluntarily. Contraction is initiated by an electrical impulse which travels down the T tubule from the cell surface. The impulse causes the sarcoplasmic reticulum to release stored calcium. In turn, the calcium initiates a change in the tropomyosin complex which allows actin and myosin to interact. During relaxation, calcium is pumped out of the sarcoplasm, actin disconnects from myosin and returns to its original position. The need for ATP to power the calcium pump is reflected in the large number of mitochondria between myofibrils.

Contracted muscle has narrower I and H bands while overstretched muscle has wider I and H bands.

Cardiac Muscle

Cardiac muscle fibers are branched and striated. A single nucleus is located in the center of the cell. Cardiac muscle fibers are joined end-to-end by specialized cell junctions known as **intercalated discs.** These junctions have numerous desmosomes to anchor adjacent cells, as well as gap junctions for communication between cells. Dyads, comprised of a T tubule and poorly developed cisternae, are located at the Z line in cardiac muscle.

Cardiac impulse conduction fibers (Purkinje fibers) are modified cardiac muscle cells. These large, light-staining cells have a central nucleus surrounded by a clear halo and peripherally-located myofibrils. Conduction fibers carry electrical impulses which regulate muscle contraction.

An extensive capillary network is present in the endomysium of cardiac muscle. Small amounts of analogous perimysium are present, but epimysium is lacking in cardiac muscle.

Cardiac muscle contracts in involuntarily fashion similar to skeletal muscle.

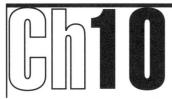

Nervous Tissue

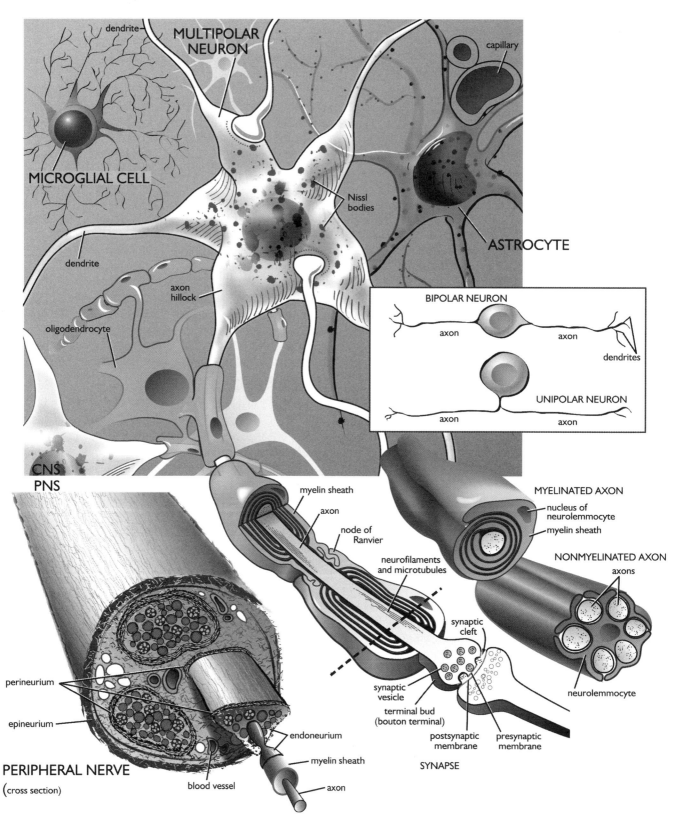

dendrite

MULTIPOLAR
NEURON

capillary

MICROGLIAL CELL

Nissl
bodies

dendrite

axon
hillock

ASTROCYTE

oligodendrocyte

BIPOLAR NEURON

axon

axon

dendrites

UNIPOLAR NEURON

axon

axon

CNS
PNS

myelin sheath

axon

node of
Ranvier

neurofilaments
and microtubules

MYELINATED AXON

nucleus of
neurolemmocyte

myelin sheath

NONMYELINATED AXON

axons

synaptic
cleft

synaptic
vesicle

neurolemmocyte

perineurium

epineurium

terminal bud
(bouton terminal)

postsynaptic
membrane

presynaptic
membrane

endoneurium

myelin sheath

PERIPHERAL NERVE

(cross section)

blood vessel

axon

SYNAPSE

Overview

- Neurons have large nuclei with prominent nucleoli.
- Nervous impulses are transmitted by flow of ions across the cell membrane of the neuron.
- The myelin sheath around axons is formed by the neurolemmocyte or oligodendrocyte.
- A synapse is comprised of neurotransmitters in synaptic vesicles, presynaptic membrane, synaptic cleft and postsynaptic membrane.
- Supporting neuroglial cells include astrocytes, oligodendrocytes and microgliocytes.
- The connective tissue of peripheral nerves is endoneurium, perineurium and epineurium.

Nervous tissue transmits electrical impulses from one part of the body to another. The nervous system is divided into the **central nervous system** (CNS), comprised of the brain and spinal cord, and the **peripheral nervous system** (PNS), which includes nerves and peripheral ganglia.

Neurons

Neurons are the predominate cell of nervous tissue. The cell membrane of neurons is polarized with a negative resting potential across the membrane. Potassium ions are present in increased concentration inside the cell while sodium and chloride ions are in higher concentration outside the cell. Potassium channels in the cell membrane allow ions to flow out of the cell down a concentration gradient, creating a net positive charge on the outside surface of the cell. The potential difference is also maintained with assistance from sodium-potassium pumps in the cell membrane which pump sodium out of the cell and potassium into the cell. When a neuron is stimulated, a small area of the membrane allows sodium ions to enter the neuron through the membrane channels. Increased sodium ions lead to a positive cytoplasmic surface of the membrane which is then said to be depolarized. After a brief refractory period during which ions cannot traverse the membrane, potassium is allowed to leave the cell and the resting membrane potential is then restored.

Individual neurons have a large nucleus with a prominent nucleolus. The cytoplasm contains **Nissl bodies** which are strongly basophilic, granular endoplasmic reticulum.

The cell body extends as a single, long **axon** or shorter **dendrites.** Dendrites receive stimuli while axons transmit neural impulses to other cells. The axon and **axon hillock,** a region of the cytoplasm where the axon leaves the cell body, are devoid of Nissl bodies. A cytoskeleton of neurofilaments and microtubules facilitates transport in the axon. A **unipolar neuron** has a single axon which rapidly branches. The cell body of a **bipolar neuron** is located in the center of its axon or at the junction of the axon and a single dendrite. **Multipolar neurons** have a single axon and several dendrites.

Axons may be surrounded by a **myelin sheath** which acts as an insulator and increases conduction rate along the axon. In the peripheral nervous system, the myelin sheath is formed by the cell membranes of the **neurolemmocyte** (Schwann cell) which wrap around the axon multiple times. The junction of two neurolemmocytes end-to-end forms an indented area called the **node of Ranvier**. A similar cell, the **oligodendrocyte,** myelinates axons in the central nervous system. Multiple axons invested by the cell membranes of the same neurolemmocyte are termed nonmyelinated.

Lipofuscin, a golden pigment linked to high cell metabolism and organelle turnover, is scattered in the cytoplasm of some neurons.

Neurosecretory vesicles containing peptides are found in many axons. An example is the stored hormones, oxytocin and antidiuretic hormone (ADH; vasopressin) in hypothalamic neurons.

Neural Synapses

Neurons contact each other at points called synapses. The cytoplasm of a presynaptic neuron has multiple **synaptic vesicles** which contain neurotransmitters such as acetylcholine, norepinephrine and dopamine. Upon stimulation of the nerve, the synaptic vesicles fuse to the **presynaptic membrane** and release their contents into the synaptic cleft between synapsing neurons. The neurotransmitters cross the cleft and bind to receptors on the **postsynaptic membrane,** initiating a neural impulse in the postsynaptic neuron.

Neuroglia

The stroma, or supporting network, of the nervous system is formed by cells rather than by connective tissue proper as in most other organs. In the central nervous system, **astrocytes, oligodendrocytes** and **microglial cell** are the principal neuroglial cells. Astrocytes have a large, round nucleus while the nucleus of oligodendrocytes is intermediate in size and microglial nuclei are the smallest. Cytoplasm of these cells is difficult to distinguish. **Ependymal cells** line the ventricles of the brain and central canal of the spinal cord. The neuroglial cells of the peripheral nervous system are the neurolemmocyte and the **ganglial gliocytes** (satellite cells; amphicytes) which surround neuron cell bodies in ganglia.

Nuclei and Ganglia

The cell bodies of neurons lie in clusters called **nuclei** in the CNS and **ganglia** in the PNS. Axons of the neurons extend to form **tracts** (CNS) or **peripheral nerves** (PNS).

Connective Tissue of Peripheral Nerves

Individual axons in a peripheral nerve are surrounded by fine connective tissue termed **endoneurium.** Epithelioid cells form the **perineurium** around a fascicle of axons. The outer surface of large nerves is covered by dense connective tissue called **epineurium.**

Receptors

Neural receptors may be **encapsulated** or **non-encapsulated.** Non-encapsulated nerve endings lack a capsular covering while encapsulated receptors are surrounded by a structure ranging from a thin covering (neuromuscular spindle) to multiple layers (lamellar receptor (Pacinian corpuscle)).

Ch11 Blood Vessels

LAYERS OF BLOOD VESSEL WALL

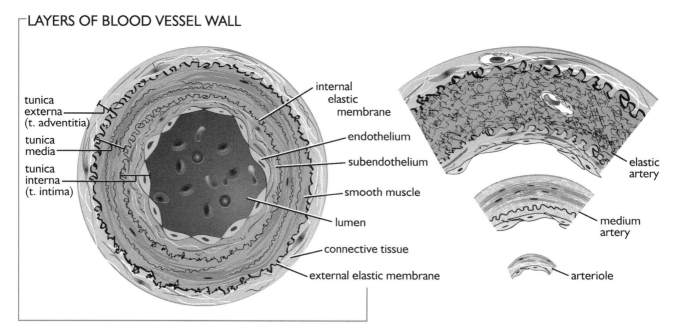

tunica externa (t. adventitia)

tunica media

tunica interna (t. intima)

internal elastic membrane

endothelium

subendothelium

smooth muscle

lumen

connective tissue

external elastic membrane

elastic artery

medium artery

arteriole

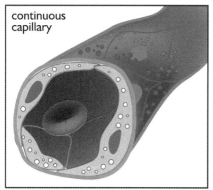

continuous capillary

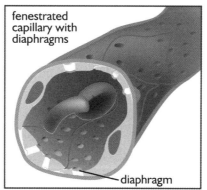

fenestrated capillary with diaphragms

diaphragm

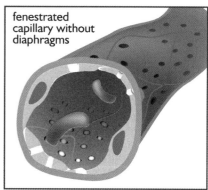

fenestrated capillary without diaphragms

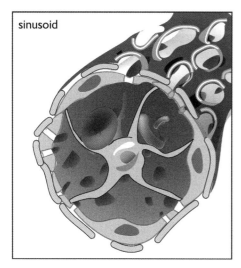

sinusoid

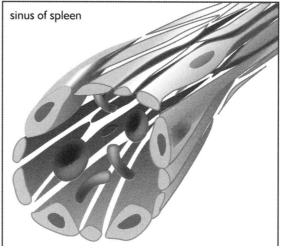

sinus of spleen

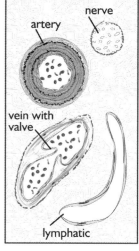

artery

nerve

vein with valve

lymphatic

Overview

- The wall of blood vessels is made up of three layers: tunica interna, tunica media and tunica externa.
- Endothelium is simple squamous epithelium which lines blood vessels.
- Arteries have abundant smooth muscle in the prominent tunica media. Elastic fibers and elastic membranes are sometimes present.
- The wall of capillaries is formed by a single layer of endothelial cells which can be continuous or fenestrated. Fenestrations may have diaphragms.
- The endothelial cells of sinusoids have large, open fenestrations while sinuses are lined by fusiform endothelial cells.
- Veins have a more prominent tunica adventitia when compared to arteries and valves are present.

Blood vessels range from large elastic arteries such as the aorta to very small capillaries. Large blood vessels transport blood around the body while exchange of nutrients and gases between the blood and surrounding tissues occurs at the capillary level.

Mural Organization of Blood Vessels

The wall of a blood vessel has various layers, depending on the size of the vessel.

The **tunica interna** (tunica intima) is adjacent to the lumen and is comprised of the endothelium, subendothelium and internal elastic membrane. **Endothelium** is simple squamous epithelium which lines blood vessels and lymphatics. Endothelial cells have characteristic pinocytotic vesicles along the cytoplasmic side of the cell membrane. In fenestrated blood vessels, the endothelial cells have transcellular pores which allow fluids and larger molecules to exit the vessel into the surrounding tissue. The **subendothelium** is fibrous connective tissue. In the deep region of the tunica interna, blood vessels may have a condensation of elastic fibers called the **internal elastic membrane.**

The **tunica media,** a mixture of smooth muscle and connective tissue, is located between the tunica interna and tunica externa. A condensation of elastic fibers, the **external elastic membrane,** is present in some vessels as an outer layer of the tunica media. Larger vessels may have their own blood and nerve supply, the **vasa vasorum** and **nervi vasorum,** represented by small blood vessels and nerves within the tunica media.

Connective tissue proper on the outer surface of the blood vessel forms the **tunica externa** (tunica adventitia). This tissue layer often blends into surrounding connective tissue.

Arteries

All mural layers described above are present in the wall of the large **elastic artery.** The tunica media of this vessel contains large amounts of elastic fibers scattered among the smooth muscle cells. The smaller **muscular artery** (medium artery) lacks elastic fibers in the tunica media but smooth muscle and a prominent internal elastic membrane remains. The wall of the **arteriole** further decreases to one or two layers of smooth muscle in the tunica media and thinner tunicae interna and externa. The internal elastic membrane is absent at the arteriolar level. A specialized arteriole, the **metarteriole,** has a discontinuous layer of smooth muscle in the tunica media. This vessel acts as a central channel through a capillary bed and controls the blood flow through the bed.

Capillaries

Capillaries have a thin wall of endothelium and a variable basement membrane. Isolated cells called **pericytes** are scattered along the capillary inside the basement membrane. These cells are undifferentiated and can become many different cells including smooth muscle.

The **continuous capillary** has no interruptions or pores in the endothelium. Tight junctions are present between cells. Continuous capillaries are found in muscle or lung.

The **fenestrated capillary** has small pores scattered throughout the endothelial cells of the vessel wall. Diaphragms, which control the size of molecules allowed to pass through the pores, may be present in some fenestrated capillaries. Fenestrated capillaries with diaphragms are found in the intestine and endocrine organs while diaphragms are lacking in the pores of renal capillary endothelial cells.

Sinusoids have a larger lumen than the fenestrated capillary described above. Large, open fenestrations of varying sizes are present in the endothelial cells. The basement membrane surrounding this type of capillary is generally incomplete. Phagocytic cells are often found either outside the endothelium or spanning the lumen of the sinusoid. Blood flow through the sinusoid is very slow. Liver and bone marrow sinusoids are an example of this type of blood vessel.

Sinuses for transport of blood in the spleen are lined by fusiform endothelial cells with intercellular gaps. Reticular fibers and an incomplete basement membrane surround the sinus. In contrast, sinuses in the lymph node transport lymph and are lined by reticular cells.

Veins

Compared to the artery of corresponding size, veins typically have a larger lumen and a thinner wall. The predominate layer of the wall of a vein is the tunica externa.

Venule walls are comprised of endothelium surrounded by a thin layer of connective tissue. **Small veins** acquire smooth muscle in the tunica media. **Medium veins** have more smooth muscle than small veins and the tunica externa is well-developed. **Large veins** have smooth muscle which is circularly arranged in the tunica media while longitudinal smooth muscle fibers are present in the tunica externa.

Veins are characterized by **valves** which extend into the lumen and prevent the back flow of blood in the vessel. Valves are leaflets of the tunica interna including endothelium and a thin connective tissue core. The vena cava and hepatic portal vein do not have valves.

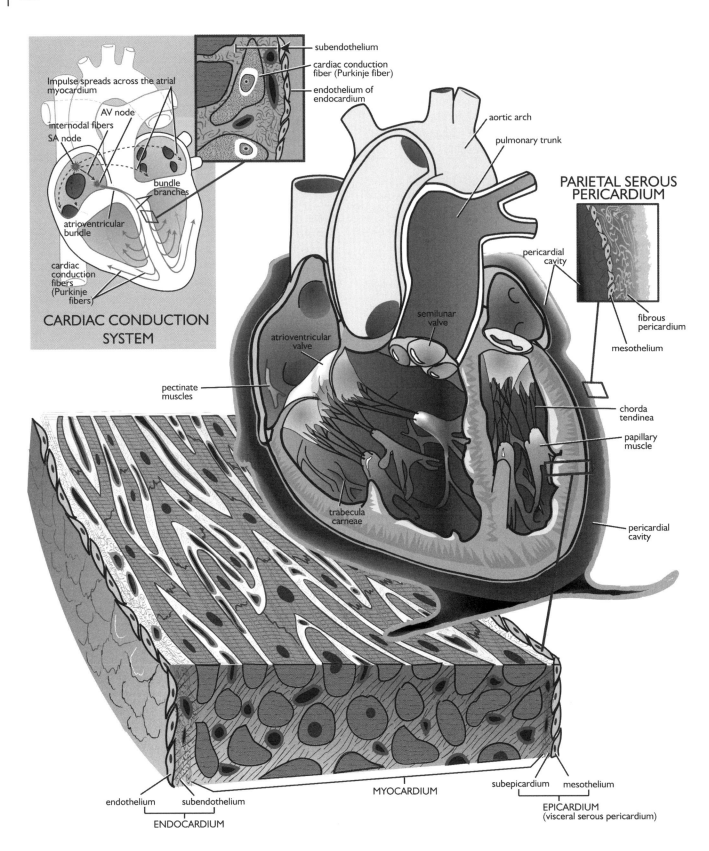

Impulse spreads across the atrial myocardium

AV node

internodal fibers

SA node

atrioventricular bundle

bundle branches

cardiac conduction fibers (Purkinje fibers)

CARDIAC CONDUCTION SYSTEM

subendothelium

cardiac conduction fiber (Purkinje fiber)

endothelium of endocardium

aortic arch

pulmonary trunk

PARIETAL SEROUS PERICARDIUM

semilunar valve

pericardial cavity

fibrous pericardium

mesothelium

atrioventricular valve

pectinate muscles

chorda tendinea

papillary muscle

trabecula carneae

pericardial cavity

endothelium   subendothelium

ENDOCARDIUM

MYOCARDIUM

subepicardium   mesothelium

EPICARDIUM (visceral serous pericardium)

Overview

- The heart has three histologic layers: endocardium, myocardium and epicardium.
- Endocardium is the inner layer of endothelium and connective tissue.
- Myocardium is thick cardiac muscle.
- Epicardium is the outer layer of mesothelial cells and connective tissue.
- Heart valves are formed by folds of endocardium.
- The cardiac skeleton is dense connective tissue which sometimes includes cartilage or bone.
- Modified cardiac muscle cells with neural properties form the nodes and the fibers of the cardiac conduction system.
- The pericardium, comprised of mesothelial layers and connective tissue, covers the heart and contains pericardial fluid within the pericardial cavity.

The heart functions as a pump to propel blood through blood vessels to the tissues and organs of the body. The mammalian heart has four chambers: two atria and two ventricles.

Mural Organization of the Heart

The **endocardium** is the inner layer of the heart and is continuous with the tunica interna of the blood vessels that enter and exit the four heart chambers. The endocardium is comprised of a lining of endothelium supported by inner and outer subendothelial layers of dense or loose connective tissue respectively. Endocardium of the atria is thicker than endocardium of the ventricles.

Cardiac muscle is the primary component of the **myocardium** which forms the middle layer of the heart wall. The cardiac muscle fibers in this layer are arranged in a spiral pattern. Cardiac muscle cells in the atria produce hormones such as atrial natriuretic polypeptide. These hormones are released into cardiac capillaries and influence blood pressure and electrolyte balance. Myocardium is thickest in the left ventricle and thinnest in the atria.

Epicardium (visceral pericardium) covers the outer surface of the heart as a single layer of mesothelial cells with underlying connective tissue. The subepicardial connective tissue contains blood vessels, nerves, and a varying amount of fat.

Endocardial-Myocardial Projections

Atrioventricular and semilunar **cardiac valves** of the heart are formed by folds of the endocardium. A dense core of connective tissue is located in the center of the valve. Lymphatics and nerves are lacking. When closed, valves prevent back flow of blood.

In the auricular portion of the atria, the innermost bundles of cardiac muscle and the overlying endocardium form the **pectinate muscles** which project into the atrial lumen. **Papillary muscles** and **trabeculae carneae** in the ventricle are also projections of myocardium with an endocardial covering. The papillary muscles anchor the connective tissue cords (chordae tendinae) from the atrioventricular-valves to the floor of the ventricles.

Cardiac Skeleton

The base of the heart where the major blood vessels enter and exit is supported by a cardiac skeleton of dense irregular connective tissue. Fibrocartilage is often present in the cardiac skeleton of dogs, while hyaline cartilage is typical in horses. Bone is present in this area in ruminants.

Cardiac Impulse Conduction System

Heart rate is controlled by the **sinoatrial node,** located in the wall of the right atrium. A wave of depolarization from the node spreads through the internodal connecting pathway to the **atrioventricular node** located at the junction of the atria and the coronary sinus near the right atrioventricular valve. Both nodes consist of modified cardiac muscle cells that are light staining and have fewer myofibrils and organelles than working cardiac myocytes.

A bundle of cardiac conduction fibers called the **atrioventricular bundle** (bundle of His) extends from the atrioventricular node through the subendocardium and divides into right and left bundle branches. The fibers of the branches ramify in the myocardium of the ventricles. **Cardiac conduction fibers** (Purkinje fibers) are wider and shorter than cardiac myocytes. They have few myofibrils and myofilaments resulting in pale cytoplasm, and a clear zone is present around the centrally located nucleus.

Blood Supply to the Heart

The layers of the heart are supplied by blood from coronary arteries that branch into a dense capillary network. The venous blood drains through venules and veins into the coronary sinus or through small cardiac veins directly through the endocardium into the heart chambers.

Pericardium

The heart is surrounded by a dense connective tissue and epithelial covering called the pericardium. The **pericardial cavity** separates the parietal and visceral layers of the pericardium, and contains a small quantity of **pericardial fluid.** The **visceral serous pericardium** (epicardium) represents the outer layer of the heart wall and is continuous at the base of the heart with the **parietal serous pericardium** on the inner surface of the pericardial sac. The **fibrous pericardium,** a dense connective tissue layer, lies beneath the mesothelial cells of the parietal serous pericardium.

Pericardial fluid is clear and contains a small amount of protein and few cells. The fluid is thought to be an ultrafiltrate produced by the visceral serous pericardium (epicardium) and drained from the pericardial space by lymphatics.

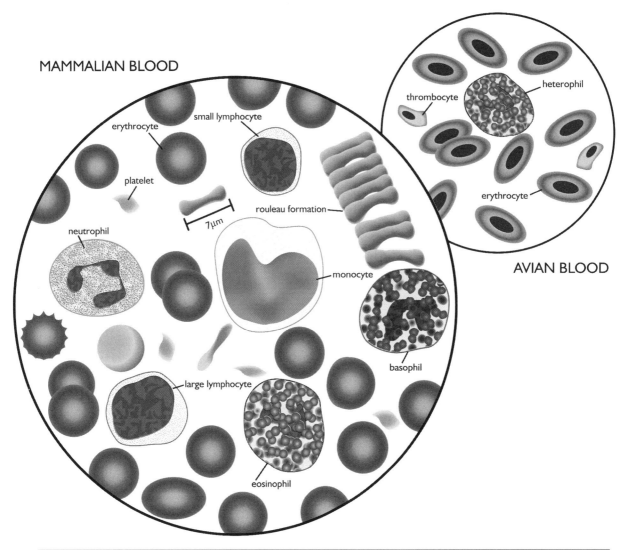

MAMMALIAN BLOOD

- erythrocyte
- small lymphocyte
- platelet
- neutrophil
- rouleau formation
- 7μm
- monocyte
- large lymphocyte
- basophil
- eosinophil

AVIAN BLOOD

- thrombocyte
- heterophil
- erythrocyte

	Lymphocyte	Monocyte	Neutrophil	Eosinophil	Basophil
Diameter (μm)	6-12	>15	12	12	12
% Cells					
Canine	20	5	71	4	1
Feline	30	5	60	5	1
Equine	35	5	55	4	1
Bovine	60	5	30	5	1
Circulating Half Life	Few months to years	Few days in blood to several months in tissue	5-10 hours	<1 up to 6 hours	6 hours to 2 weeks once in tissues
Nuclear shape	Round	Indented	3-5 lobes	2 lobes	Segmented
Nuclear:cytoplas - mic ratio	High	Low	Moderate	Moderate	Moderate
Granules (Wright's stain)	-	-	Pale reddish blue	Pink to orange	Dark blue to black

Overview

- Erythrocytes are anucleate, biconcave disks which transport oxygen and carbon dioxide.
- Neutrophils have pale granules and a lobated nucleus.
- Eosinophils have eosinophilic granules while basophils have basophilic granules.
- Lymphocytes have a round nucleus with a thin rim of cytoplasm and no granules.
- Monocytes have an indented nucleus and numerous cytoplasmic vacuoles of varying size.
- Platelets are fragments of megakaryocytes. Platelets and thrombocytes function in blood clotting.

Mammalian blood is composed of plasma, cells and platelets. Blood cells and platelets are produced in the bone marrow. Plasma is the fluid component of blood.

Erythrocytes

The **erythrocyte,** or red blood cell (RBC), is the most numerous cell in blood. The mammalian cell is a biconcave disk which is devoid of a nucleus and organelles and measures 4-7 micrometers in diameter. In contrast, erythrocytes from avians and many lower species are ovoid and contain numerous organelles including a nucleus. Spectrin, a membrane protein, helps maintain the shape of mammalian erythrocytes. The average lifespan of an erythrocyte is 120 days.

Characteristics of erythrocytes, such as variation in size **(anisocytosis)** or shape **(poikilocytosis),** can indicate certain diseases. **Rouleau** formation occurs when erythrocytes adhere to one another in cellular stacks. Shrinkage of the cell may result in erythrocytes with spines and is an artifact of drying called crenation.

Howell-Jolly bodies are fragments of nuclear material which stain as dark purple dots in the cytoplasm of erythrocytes from dogs and cats. With the use of vital stains, inclusions of oxidized hemoglobin called **Heinz bodies** can also be demonstrated in feline erythrocytes.

The cytoplasm of erythrocytes contains hemoglobin and various enzymes. **Hemoglobin** is a large protein bound to heme, which contains iron. The protein portion of hemoglobin releases carbon dioxide while the iron portion binds oxygen in the lung. Upon reaching tissues with low oxygen concentration, the converse occurs - oxygen is released and carbon dioxide is bound for transport. Enzymes in the cytoplasm of erythrocytes include carbonic anhydrase which facilitates for formation of carbonic acid from carbon dioxide and water. Carbonic acid is dissociated to form bicarbonate which is then transported to the lungs by erythrocytes, released, and exhaled.

Leukocytes

Leukocytes are round, nucleated blood cells. Migrating leukocytes can leave circulating blood and enter surrounding tissues by diapedesing between endothelial cells. Granulocytes have cytoplasmic granules which are not present in agranulocytes.

The nucleus of **polymorphonuclear granulocytes** is lobate. This class of leukocytes includes the neutrophil, eosinophil and basophil. **Neutrophils** have pale, granules which are difficult to discern. The nucleus is lobate and ery-

throcytes from females may have a small secondary nuclear appendage called a **Barr body** which represents one of the X chromosomes. The neutrophil is phagocytic and readily migrates to the site of acute infection. Avian **heterophils** are analogous to mammalian neutrophils except that they have eosinophilic granules. **Eosinophils** have characteristic large, eosinophilic granules in the cytoplasm. The nucleus of the eosinophil is bilobed. Eosinophils phagocytize antigen-antibody complexes and are increased in number in parasitic infestations. **Basophils** have basophilic-staining granules which contain heparin and histamine similar to mast cell granules. The granules can obscure the segmented nucleus of the basophil which is involved in the regulation of inflammation.

Mononuclear agranulocytes have a single, round to indented nucleus with no prominent cytoplasmic granules. This class of cells includes the lymphocyte and monocyte. The dense nucleus of the **lymphocyte** is surrounded by a thin rim of cytoplasm with fine lysosomal granules. Small to large lymphocytes are further classified with immunocytochemistry as B cells, T cells, or NK (natural killer cells). Plasma cells represent the fully differentiated lymphocyte. The **monocyte** has an indented nucleus and a greater cytoplasmic:nuclear ratio than the lymphocyte. The cytoplasm of monocytes has vacuoles of varying size. Monocytes are the largest leukocyte and are phagocytic cells. Macrophages are monocytes which have migrated into tissue and are characteristically present in chronic inflammation.

Platelets and Thrombocytes

Platelets are small fragments of megakaryocytes. The platelet lacks a nucleus. Microtubules in the periphery of the cytoplasm help maintain the shape of the platelet. An **open canalicular system** creates channels that increase surface area for exchange with surrounding plasma. Calcium and hormones localize in a **dense tubular system** in the center of the platelet. Platelets play a role in the formation of blood clots by adhering to breaks in the endothelium of damaged blood vessels and to other platelets thus forming an aggregate at the time of clotting.

Thrombocytes are found in the blood of avians and lower vertebrates. The thrombocyte is nucleated and has a clear cytoplasm with small red granules. Thrombocytes function in blood clotting, are phagocytic, and develop from erythrocytic precursors instead of forming from the megakaryocyte.

Plasma

The fluid component of blood is **plasma** which is composed of water with a small percentage of proteins, inorganic salts and other organic compounds including amino acids, hormones and lipoproteins. Plasma proteins include albumin, alpha-, beta- and gamma-globulins, and fibrinogen. If plasma is allowed to clot and the clot is removed, the residual fluid is **serum.**

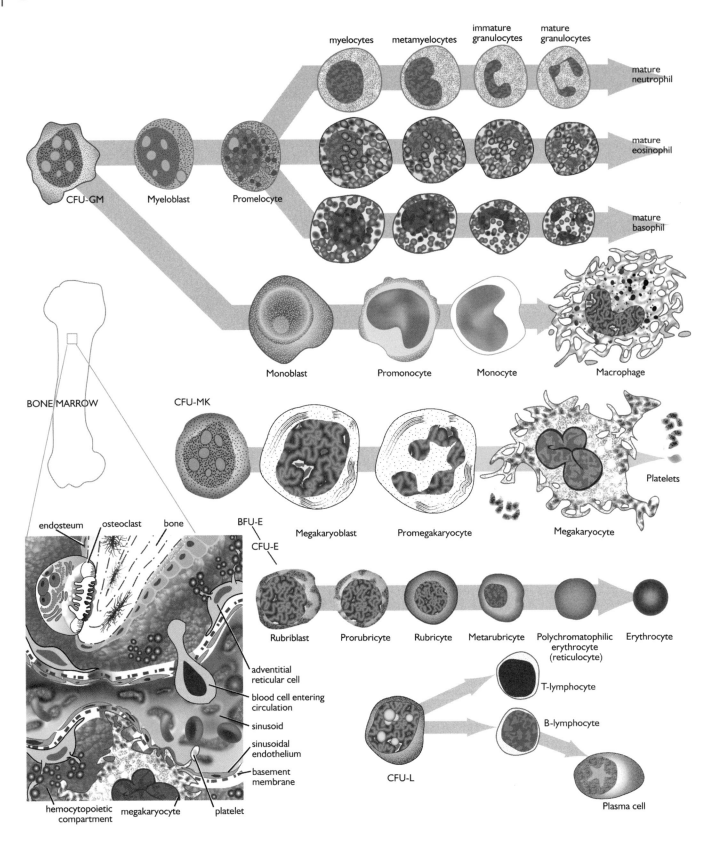

myelocytes   metamyelocytes   immature granulocytes   mature granulocytes   mature neutrophil

mature eosinophil

mature basophil

CFU-GM   Myeloblast   Promelocyte

Monoblast   Promonocyte   Monocyte   Macrophage

BONE MARROW

CFU-MK

CFU-MK

Megakaryoblast   Promegakaryocyte   Megakaryocyte   Platelets

endosteum   osteoclast   bone

BFU-E

CFU-E

Rubriblast   Prorubricyte   Rubricyte   Metarubricyte   Polychromatophilic erythrocyte (reticulocyte)   Erythrocyte

adventitial reticular cell

blood cell entering circulation

sinusoid

sinusoidal endothelium

basement membrane

T-lymphocyte

B-lymphocyte

CFU-L

hemocytopoietic compartment   megakaryocyte   platelet

Plasma cell

Overview

- Red bone marrow actively produces blood cells while yellow bone marrow is primarily adipose tissue.
- The erythrocytic cell series progresses from the rubriblast through the prorubricyte, rubricyte, metarubricyte, and polychromatophilic erythrocyte to the mature erythrocyte.
- The leukocytic cell series includes the myeloblast, promyelocyte, myelocyte, metamyelocyte, immature granulocyte (band cell), and mature granulocyte.
- Megakaryocytes release fragments of their cytoplasm into the blood circulation as platelets.
- Blood cell formation can be intramedullary or extramedullary.
- Uncommitted stem cells give rise to committed stem cells which differentiate into various blood cells lines.
- New blood cells are released from the hemocytopoietic compartment of bone marrow into the bone marrow sinusoid.

Bone marrow is found in the medullary cavity of long bones and the spongy bone of flat bones. Red bone marrow is highly cellular and is actively engaged in blood cell and platelet formation (hemocytopoiesis and thrombocytopoiesis) while yellow marrow is primarily adipose tissue. The hemocytopoietic compartment of bone marrow contains blood cells in various stages of development, megakaryocytes, macrophages, and supporting reticular cells which are arranged in cords. The vascular compartment includes the sinusoids. Bone marrow is separated from adjacent bone by the endosteum.

Cells of Bone Marrow

The **erythrocytic (red) cell series** progresses from the rubriblast through the prorubricyte, rubricyte, metarubricyte, and polychromatophilic erythrocyte to the mature erythrocyte. The **rubriblast** has a euchromatic nucleus with prominent nucleoli and a basophilic cytoplasm. Less euchromatin, no nucleoli and a basophilic cytoplasm are typical features of the **prorubricyte**. The **rubricyte** has a heterochromatic nucleus with blue to bluish-red cytoplasm. A dense, small heterochromatic nucleus is characteristic of the **metarubricyte** which is no longer capable of mitosis. Cytoplasm is bluish in the polychromatophilic erythrocyte (reticulocyte) and a nucleus is absent. Once mature, the erythrocyte cytoplasm loses its blue color and is pink to orange when stained with Wright's stain.

The **leukocytic (white) cell series** includes the myeloblast, promyelocyte, myelocyte, metamyelocyte, immature granulocyte (band cell), and mature granulocyte. The **myeloblast** has a euchromatic nucleus, prominent nucleoli and pale blue cytoplasm. The nucleus of the **promyelocyte,** like the prorubricyte, is less euchromatic and no nucleoli are seen. Primary granules are present in the pale blue cytoplasm of the promyelocyte. At the **myelocyte** stage, heterochromatin increases in the nucleus and secondary granules, which are characteristic for each cell series, appear in the cytoplasm. The **metamyelocyte** has an indented nucleus and is no longer capable of mitosis. The nucleus of the **immature granulocyte** (band cell) is further indented to form a C- or S-shaped structure without constrictions. With continued differentiation, the **mature granulocyte** nucleus has distinct segments characteristic of the cell type.

In contrast to the multinucleated osteoclast also found in bone marrow, **megakaryocytes** are large cells with a single polyploid nucleus. These cells, located adjacent to the wall of the sinusoid, release membrane-bounded fragments of their cytoplasm into circulating blood as platelets. Megakaryocytes are absent in avians and lower vertebrates.

Macrophages in bone marrow have many functions including association with differentiating lymphocytes and phagocytosis of nuclei released from erythrocytes during differentiation.

Blood Cell Formation

Blood cell development occurs at different sites in the body. Prenatally and during certain diseases, blood cells are formed outside the bone marrow **(extramedullary hemocytopoiesis)** in the yolk sac, liver, and spleen. **Medullary hemocytopoiesis** is the formation of blood cells within the bone marrow.

Colony-forming units (CFU) are cells identified through tissue culture studies and thought to be precursors of specific cell lines. **Uncommitted hemocytopoietic stem cells** (CFU-S) can reproduce and give rise to committed stem cells. The **committed stem cells** continue to develop into specific cell lines and include the erythrocytic, leukocytic, and lymphocytic stem cells. **CFU-GM** are the stem cells for precursor cells of monocytes, neutrophils, eosinophils, and basophils. **CFU-MK** are the stem cells for megakaryocytes and **CFU-E** are the stem cells for erythrocytes. The lymphoid stem cell divides to form B and T progenitor cells. The B cell goes through initial differentiation in the cloacal bursa in avians or a bursa-equivalent area, the bone marrow, in mammals, while the T cell begins differentiation in the thymus. Immunocompetent B and T cells then migrate to secondary lymphoid organs such as the tonsil, lymph nodes and spleen.

Certain growth factors stimulate the development of hematopoietic stem cells. These growth factors include erythropoietin, granulopoietin, thrombopoietin, and interleukins.

Release of New Blood Cells into Circulation

Mature blood cells leave the hemocytopoietic compartment by crossing the sparse basement membrane of the sinusoidal endothelium and exiting the bone marrow through transient fenestrations in the endothelial cells.

Hypophysis Cerebri and Epiphysis Cerebri

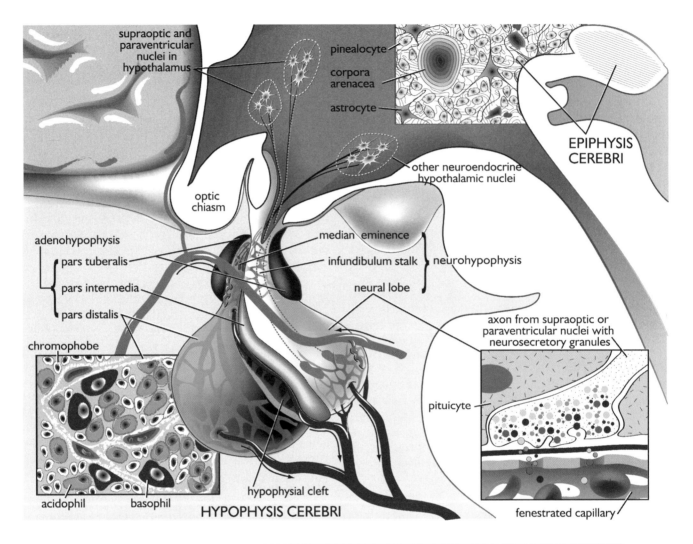

supraoptic and paraventricular nuclei in hypothalamus

pinealocyte

corpora arenacea

astrocyte

other neuroendocrine hypothalamic nuclei

EPIPHYSIS CEREBRI

optic chiasm

median eminence

infundibulum stalk

neural lobe

neurohypophysis

adenohypophysis

pars tuberalis

pars intermedia

pars distalis

chromophobe

axon from supraoptic or paraventricular nuclei with neurosecretory granules

pituicyte

acidophil   basophil

hypophysial cleft

HYPOPHYSIS CEREBRI

fenestrated capillary

Chromophils of the Pars Distalis				
Chromophil subclass	Cell	Hormone	Releasing factor	Target organ
Acidophils	Somatotropes	Somatotropin (STH)	SRH -release Somatostatin -inhibit	Increase metabolism of most cells; skeletal growth
	Lactotropes	Prolactin	PRF -release PIF -inhibit	Mammary gland (crop in some birds)
Basophils	Thyrotopes	Thyrotropin (TSH)	TRH -release	Thyroid
	Gonadotropes	Luteinizing hormone (LH) Follicle stimulating hormone (FSH)	GnRH -release	Testes and ovaries
	Corticotropes	Adrenocorticotropic hormone (ACTH) β-lipotropin (β-LPH)	CRH -release	Adrenal Hypophysis for β−endorphin production
	Melanotropes	Melanocyte stimulating hormone (MSH)	MIF -inhibit	Skin

Overview

- The hypophysis cerebri includes the adenohypophysis (pars distalis, pars tuberalis and pars intermedia) and neurohypophysis (median eminence, infundibular stalk and neural lobe).
- Cells of the pars distalis are chromophobes, acidophils and basophils. Based on hormones produced by the cells, the acidophils can be further subdivided into somatotropes and lactotropes while basophils can be classed as thyrotropes, gonadotropes or corticotropes.
- Axons of the neurohypophysis store neurosecretory granules containing oxytocin and ADH.
- The hypophysial portal system transports hypothalamic secretions to cells in the pars distalis where the secretions influence hormone release.
- Pinealocytes of the epiphysis cerebri produce melatonin and serotonin.
- Corpora arenacea are calcified intercellular deposits in the epiphysis cerebri.

The hypophysis cerebri (pituitary) and epiphysis cerebri (pineal) are endocrine organs which are closely associated with the brain.

General Organization of the Hypophy- sis Cerebri

The hypophysis includes the **adenohypophysis** and **neurohypophysis.** The adenohypophysis consists of the **pars distalis, pars tuberalis** and **pars intermedia.** The neurohypophysis is comprised of the median eminence, infundibular stalk and neural lobe (lobus nervosus; pars nervosa).

Structure of the Adenohypophysis

The cells of the pars distalis include **chromophils** which have acidophilic or basophilic cytoplasm and **chromophobes** with cytoplasm which stains minimally. Chromophobes represent about 50% of the cells in the pars distalis and are thought to be resting chromophils. **Acidophils,** which make up about 40% of the pars distalis cells, can be further subdivided into **somatotropes** (alpha cells) which produce somatotropin and **lactotropes** (epsilon cells) which secrete prolactin. **Basophils** are limited to about 10% of the cell population and include thyrotropes, gonadotropes and corticotropes. **Thyrotropes** (beta cells) produce thyrotropin, **gonadotropes** (delta cells) produce luteinizing hormone and follicle stimulating hormone, and **corticotropes** secrete adrenocorticotrophic hormone and beta-lipotropin. Immunohistochemistry is required to recognize specific subclasses of acidophils or basophils.

The cells of the pars tuberalis are weakly basophilic. Their function is uncertain but they have numerous melatonin receptors and may play a role in seasonal reproduction.

Melanotropes which produce melanocyte-stimulating hormone are the primary cell of the pars intermedia. The pars intermedia is separated from the pars distalis by the **hypophysial cleft.**

A fine stroma of connective tissue supports the parenchymal cells of the adenohypophysis. Stellate and follicular cells are interspersed between the secretory cells. The blood supply is well developed and consists of capillary beds typical of an endocrine organ.

Structure of the Neurohypophysis

A ventral evagination of nervous tissue from the hypothalamus forms the neurohypophysis. The **median eminence** continues as the **infundibulum stalk** which extends ventrally to form the **neural lobe** (lobus nervosus; pars nervosa). Axons projecting from neuron cell bodies in the supraoptic and paraventricular nuclei of the hypothalamus make up most of the neural lobe. The axons contain **neurosecretory granules** (Herring bodies) which are membrane-bounded vesicles containing the stored form of **oxytocin** and **antidiuretic hormone** (ADH; vasopressin). **Neurophysins,** proteins which are co-synthesized with the hormones in the cell body, are also present in the granules. **Pituicytes** are modified astrocytes which form a supportive framework around the axons and the capillary bed of the neurohypophysis.

Hypothalmo-adenohypophysial System

The hypothalmo-adenohypophysial system includes **neuroendocrine cells** of the hypothalmus and the **hypophysial portal system.**

In the median eminence near the base of the brain, arteries form the first capillary bed of the portal system. Secretions from the hypothalamic neuroendocrine cells enter blood circulation at the primary capillary bed and travel through the portal venules in the pars tuberalis. The hypothalamic secretions are released at the second capillary bed in the pars distalis to target adjacent hypophysial cells. The secretions either stimulate or inhibit the release of hormones from the target cells. Released hormones then enter the second capillary bed and the hormone-rich blood exits the hypophysis through draining venules.

In contrast, in the neural lobe, a single capillary bed transports the hormones released from the axons.

Structure of the Epiphysis Cerebri

Pinealocytes, the primary cells of the epiphysis cerebri or pineal, are large basophilic cells with round nuclei. **Synaptic ribbons** in the cytoplasm of pinealocytes increase in number during dark periods of a light-dark cycle but are of uncertain function. The synaptic ribbons are visible with electron microscopy and are comprised of dense rod-like profiles surrounded by vesicles. **Astrocytes** interdigitate between the pinealocytes and capillaries. Intercellular calcium deposits called **corpora arenacea** are associated with aging but do not seem to affect glandular function. The epiphysis cerebri is surrounded by a capsule of pia mater. This light-sensitive endocrine organ is responsible for the production of melatonin and serotonin.

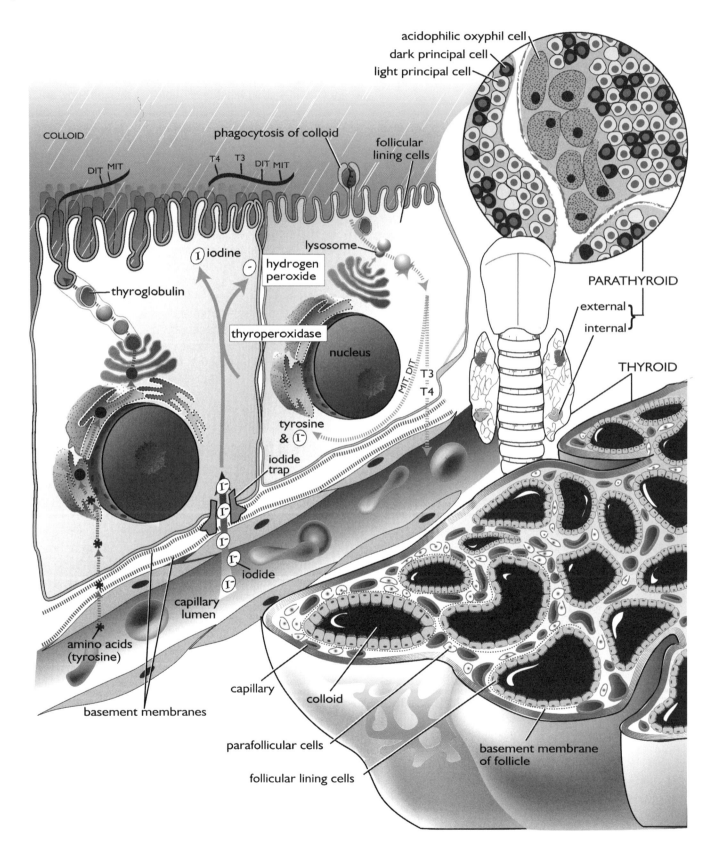

Overview

- Thyroid follicles are lined by follicular lining cells which produce thyroid hormones.
- Colloid, the stored form of thyroid hormone, is located in the center of the follicle.
- Parafollicular cells, located outside the follicular lining epithelium, produce calcitonin.
- Follicular lining cells process iodide and proteins to form thyroglobulin which is stored as the colloid. The colloid is then mobilized and metabolized to T_3 and T_4 which is released into blood circulation.
- Principal cells of the parathyroid produce PTH.
- Oxyphil cells are large, pale cells of unknown function which are present in parathyroid glands of the ox, horse and man.

The thyroid and parathyroid gland are endocrine glands which are located in the cervical region, ventral and lateral to the trachea.

Structure of the Thyroid

Parenchyma of the thyroid is arranged in spherical follicles which are surrounded by a dense capillary network. The size of the follicles varies with activity.

Epithelium of the follicles consists of **follicular lining cells** which vary from squamous to columnar in shape. The lining cells are acidophilic with numerous cytoplasmic secretory vesicles, a basal nucleus and microvilli on the apical surface. An acidophilic gel-like material called colloid is located in the center of the follicle. Colloid is the stored precursor of thyroid hormone which functions in cellular energy metabolism, growth and differentiation.

Parafollicular cells (C cells) are located outside the follicular lining epithelium and do not extend to the lumen of the follicle. The parafollicular cells are lighter staining than follicular lining cells. Parafollicular cells produce calcitonin which decreases blood calcium.

The thyroid gland is surrounded by a connective tissue capsule which extends as fine septa between the follicles. The septa contain lymphatics, nerves and a rich blood supply typical of an endocrine organ.

Synthesis and Storage of Thyroid Hormone

Under the influence of thyroid stimulating hormone (TSH) from the hypophysis cerebi, the follicular lining epithelial cells remove circulating iodide from blood in adjacent capillaries. The iodide is concentrated and oxidized to iodine within the epithelial cells by a peroxidase located at the microvilli. Concurrently, polypeptides are synthesized and glycosylated to form thyroglobulin in the epithelial cells. The thyroglobulin is transported to the colloid where it is then iodinated to form mono- and diiodotyrosine which are the building blocks of tri-iodothyronine (T_3) and tetraiodothyronine (T_4; thyroxine).

Mobilization of Thyroid Hormone

Mobilization of thyroid hormone is also regulated by TSH. The follicular epithelial cells form large apical pseudopods under TSH stimulation. Colloid becomes vesicular around the edges and intracellular colloid droplets increase as thyroglobulin is phagocytosed. Secondary lysosomes fuse with the thyroglobulin and iodinated molecules are cleaved. Iodinated tyrosine is recycled into iodide and tyrosine for future use within the cell and T_3 and T_4 are released across the basal cell membrane into blood circulation.

Structure of the Parathyroid Glands

External parathyroid glands are located at the cranial pole of the thyroid while internal parathyroids are embedded within the thyroid tissue at the caudal pole. The external gland is absent in birds and pigs. Accessory parathyroid tissue in other locations is common.

A thin connective tissue capsule surrounds the parathyroid gland and often blends with connective tissue of the nearby thyroid. Fine septa extend from the capsule into the parenchyma and contain the rich endocrine blood supply.

The cells of the parathyroid are arranged in clusters or cords between the septa. The **principal cells** (chief cells) are polygonal cells with a round nucleus. Principal cells can be classified as light or dark sub populations which are thought to be different physiologic states of the same cell. The **light principal cell** (water clear cell) is most common and appears to be inactive. Cell membranes of the light principal cell are prominent and the cytoplasm contains abundant glycogen or lipofuscin in some species. **Dark principal cells** actively produce parathyroid hormone (PTH) which increases blood calcium levels. PTH acts by increasing mobilization of calcium from bone, increasing calcium absorption in the intestines, and reducing calcium loss in the urine.

Scattered large, acidophilic cells called **oxyphil cells** are present in the parathyroid of the ox, horse and man. The function of the oxyphil cell is unknown.

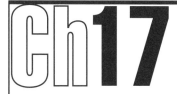

Zones and Hormones of the Suprarenal Cortex

Cortical zone	Hormone	Regulator	Target organ
Zona glomerulosa	Mineralocorticoids (aldosterone)	angiotensin adrenocorticotropic hormone (ACTH)	distal convoluted tubule of kidney
Zona fasiculata	Glucocorticoid production (cortisol and corticosterone) Some androgens and estrogens	ACTH	Glucocorticoids - general metabolism- both anabolic and catabolic Androgens and estrogens - reproductive organs
Zona reticularis	Androgens (dehydroepiandrosterone and androstenedione) and estrogens Some glucocorticoids		

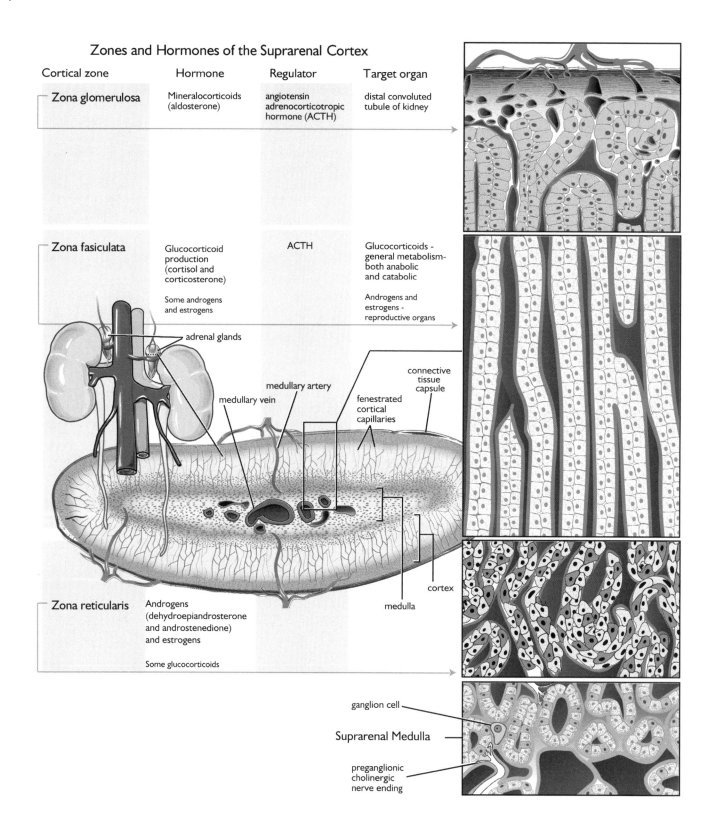

adrenal glands

medullary vein

medullary artery

fenestrated cortical capillaries

connective tissue capsule

cortex

medulla

ganglion cell

Suprarenal Medulla

preganglionic cholinergic nerve ending

Overview

- The zones of the suprarenal cortex are the zona glomerlosa, zona fasiculata, and zona reticularis. Some species also have a zona intermedia.
- Mineralocorticoids are produced by the cells of the zona glomerulosa. Glucocorticoids are primarily produced by the cells of the zona fasiculata along with minimal androgens and estrogens while the converse is true for the zona reticularis.
- Medullary endocrine cells have secretory granules containing the catecholamines, epinephrine and norepinephrine.
- Cortical blood vessels include both fenestrated capillaries with diaphragms and non-fenestrated vessels that pass through to the medulla.
- The suprarenal medulla has a dual blood supply which provides both fresh blood and blood rich in adrenocorticosteroids from the suprarenal cortex.

The suprarenal glands (adrenal glands) are located adjacent to the cranial medial border of the kidneys and represent two distinct endocrine tissues. The outer cortex secretes steroid hormones while the medulla produces catecholamines. Hormone production in each of these two regions of the gland is regulated independently.

The gland is surrounded by a dense fibrous connective tissue capsule. Connective tissue trabecula extend into the parenchyma from the capsule and a fine stroma supports the glandular cells.

Suprarenal Cortex

Cells of the suprarenal cortex are arranged in cords or glomerular structures. The cortical cells have increased smooth endoplasmic reticulum and mitochondria which both have enzymes for steroidogenesis. Cholesterol, a precursor of the steroid hormones, is stored in the numerous cytoplasmic lipid droplets. When the cortical cells are appropriately stimulated, cholesterol is released from the droplets and used in the synthesis of glucocorticoids, mineralocorticoids and androgens.

Three zones of cortical cells can be identified in most species and a fourth is present in horses and carnivores. The **zona glomerulosa** (or zona arcuata in some species) is the outer zone adjacent to the capsule. Cuboidal to columnar cells in the zona glomerulosa are arranged in glomeruli (ruminant) or curved cords (zona arcuata of the dog, cat, pig and horse). Mineralocorticoids are produced by the zona glomerulosa cells under the influence of hormones from the kidney (angiotensin II) and hypophysis cerebri (ACTH).

The **zona intermedia,** a zone of small undifferentiated cells, is present between the zona glomerulosa and zona fasiculata in horses and carnivores.

Cells of the **zona fasiculata** are cuboidal and have characteristic foamy cytoplasm due to a large amount of lipid. The zona fasiculata is the widest of the cortical zones.

Adjacent to the suprarenal medulla, the **zona reticularis** is the innermost zone of the cortex. Cells of the zona reticularis are less foamy than the cells of the zona fasiculata.

Glucocorticoids and a small amount of androgens and estrogens are produced by cells in the zona fasiculata. Conversely, more androgens and estrogens and a small amount of glucocorticoids are produced in the zona reticularis. Cells in both the zona fasiculata and zona reticularis are regulated by ACTH.

Suprarenal Medulla

The **medullary endocrine cells** (chromaffin cells) of the suprarenal medulla are modified postganglionic sympathetic neurons. During development, these cells lose their axons and dendrites and become secretory. In animals, two populations of endocrine cells are recognized based on the catecholamines present in cytoplasmic membrane-bounded dense granules. The granules contain one of the catecholamines, **epinephrine** or **norepinephrine,** along with **chromogranins** which serve as binding proteins for the catecholamines. **Epinephrine cells,** which stain lightly with chromaffin stains, represent the majority of medullary cells. **Norepinephrine cells** are fewer and stain darker with the chromaffin technique than epinephrine cells. The endocrine cells are directly innervated by preganglionic sympathetic cholinergic fibers which release aceylcholine to directly control cell secretory activity. Occasional scattered **ganglion cells** are present in the medulla.

Blood Supply to the Suprarenal Gland

Afferent arteries in the capsule of the suprarenal gland branch to supply the cortex or continue directly into the medulla. One set of cortical blood vessels is comprised of fenestrated capillaries with diaphragms. Adrenocortico- tropic hormones enter blood in the capillaries from adjacent cortical cells. A separate set of arteries passes directly through the cortex without branching and provides fresh external blood supply to the medulla. Thus the medullary cells have a dual blood supply.

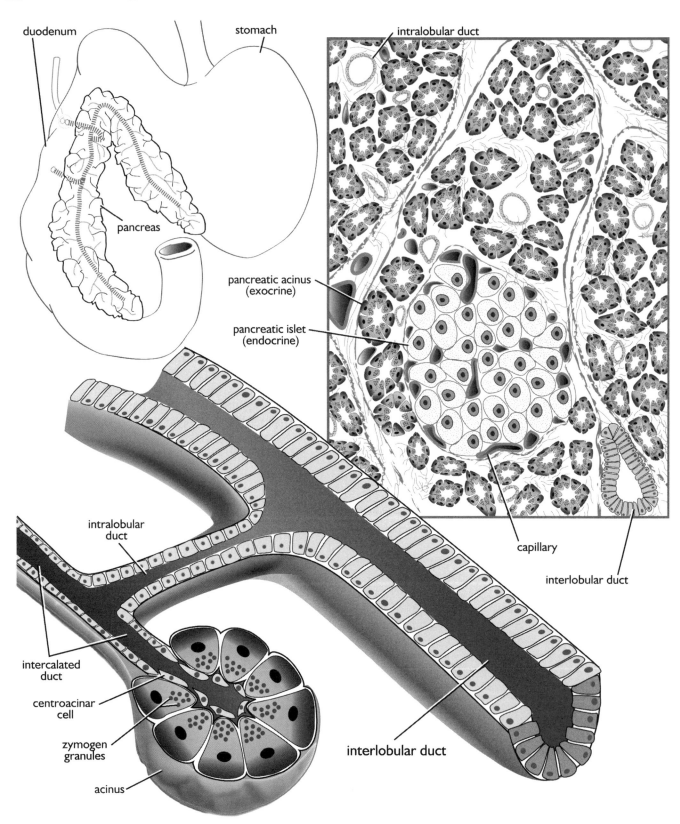

Ch18 Pancreas

duodenum

stomach

pancreas

intralobular duct

pancreatic acinus
(exocrine)

pancreatic islet
(endocrine)

capillary

interlobular duct

intralobular
duct

intercalated
duct

centroacinar
cell

zymogen
granules

acinus

interlobular duct

Overview

- Endocrine pancreatic islets are scattered among exocrine secretory units.
- In the islets, the A cell produces glucagon, the B cell produces insulin, and the D cell produces somatostatin and vasoactive intestinal peptide.
- The cells of the exocrine secretory units are arranged in acini which empty into a duct system leading to the small intestine.
- Exocrine acinar cells produce trypsinogen and chymotrypsinogen.
- Centroacinar cells are lining epithelial cells of the intercalated ducts which extend into the lumen of the exocrine acinus. The centroacinar cells are a distinguishing feature of the exocrine pancreas.

The pancreas is located in the mesentery adjacent to the duodenum. The organ is surrounded by thin connective tissue which extends between lobules of the parenchyma. Endocrine **pancreatic islets** are scattered among exocrine secretory units.

Pancreatic Islets

The pancreatic islets (islets of Langerhans) are clusters of endocrine cells. Four different cell types can only be distinguished with histochemistry or transmission electron microscopy (TEM). Cells of the islets are connected by gap junctions to facilitate intercellular communication. Numerous fenestrated capillaries with diaphragms are located in the fine connective tissue between cells.

The **A cell** (alpha cell) has dense cytoplasmic granules surrounded by a halo which is visible with TEM. This type of cell secretes glucagon, cholecystokinin, gastric inhibitory protein and ACTH-endorphin. Glucagon stimulates glycogen breakdown which increases blood glucose levels. Cholecystokinin stimulates contraction of the gallbladder and release of pancreatic enzymes. Gastric inihibitory protein inhibits the secretion of gastric acid and pepsin and stimulates the release of insulin in the pancreas.

The **B cell** (beta cell) is the most numerous cell in the islet. Cytoplasmic granules are surrounded by a halo as in the A cell, but the granules are less dense or even crystalloid in appearance. Proinsulin is produced in the granular endoplasmic reticulum of the B cell and transported to the Golgi apparatus where it is released in membrane-bounded secretory granules. During transport from the Golgi apparatus to the cell surface, the proinsulin is converted to insulin. The secretory vesicles fuse with the cell membrane, insulin is released, and the hormone enters nearby capillaries. Insulin stimulates both the conversion of glucose to fat throughout the body and the synthesis of glycogen in tissues such as liver and muscle. The overall effect of insulin is to decrease blood glucose.

D cells (delta cells) have large, pale cytoplasmic granules. Somatostatin and vasoactive intestinal peptide (VIP) are the principle products of the D cell. Somatostatin inhibits insulin and glucagon secretion in a local paracrine fashion. VIP induces glycogen break down and stimulates gastrointestinal fluid secretion.

Other islet cells include the **pancreatic polypeptide cells** (PP cells; F cells) and the **G cell.** Pancreatic polypeptide hormone increases glycogenolysis and regulates gastrointestinal activity. Gastrin from the G cell stimulates production of gastric acid by parietal cells in the stomach.

Exocrine Secretory Units of the Pancreas

The compound tubuloacinar secretory units of the exocrine pancreas surround the endocrine islets. Pyramidal-shaped secretory cells are arranged in acini which are connected to a duct system. The acinar cells each have a spherical nucleus, prominent granular endoplasmic reticulum, and numerous mitochondria in the basal region of the cell. The apical portion of the cell is filled with secretory vesicles called **zymogen granules** which represent the stored form of pancreatic enzymes.

The initial portion of the exocrine duct system, known as the **intercalated duct,** is lined by flattened simple cuboidal epithelial cells. The epithelium extends into the lumen of the acinus where the lining cells are termed **centroacinar cells.** The presence of centroacinar cells distinguishes the secretory units of exocrine pancreas from similar appearing secretory units of serous salivary glands. Epithelial cells of the intercalated ducts produce bicarbonate and water which is added to the exocrine pancreatic secretions.

The intercalated duct connects with the **intralobular duct** which is lined by simple cuboidal epithelium. Larger **interlobular ducts** are located in the connective tissue between lobules and are lined with simple columnar epithelium. The interlobular ducts empty into the pancreatic duct or accessory pancreatic duct, depending on the location within the gland and the species.

Pancreatic enzymes associated with the cells of the exocrine acini include the proenzymes, trypsinogen and chymotrypsinogen. These enzymes are produced in the acinar cells and stored in secretory vesicles in an inactive form. Following secretion into the small intestine, the enzymes are activated. Trypsinogen is converted to active trypsin by enterokinase. Active trypsin, in turn, activates chymotrypsinogen to active chymotrypsin. Both active enzymes digest proteins and peptides into smaller peptides.

Two other important pancreatic enzymes are pancreatic lipase and amylase. Lipase breaks down lipids for absorption across the intestinal epithelium while amylase hydrolyzes carbohydrates.

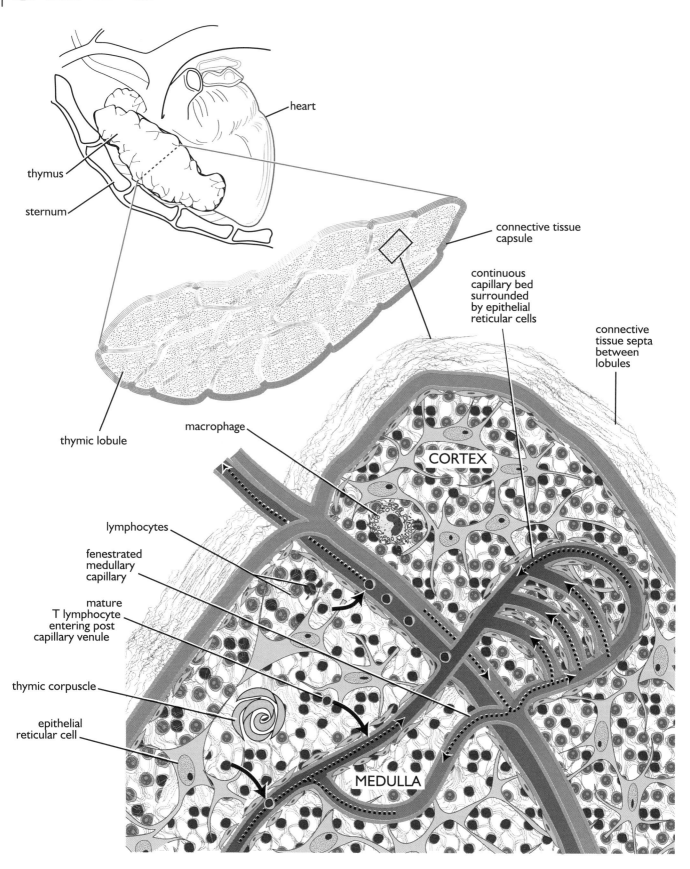

heart

thymus

sternum

connective tissue capsule

continuous capillary bed surrounded by epithelial reticular cells

connective tissue septa between lobules

thymic lobule

macrophage

CORTEX

lymphocytes

fenestrated medullary capillary

mature T lymphocyte entering post capillary venule

thymic corpuscle

epithelial reticular cell

MEDULLA

Overview

- The thymus plays a role in T lymphocyte maturation.
- Lobules of the thymus have a dark-staining cortex and a lighter-staining medulla.
- Epithelial reticular cells form the framework of the organ.
- Thymocytes (developing T lymphocytes) mature within the epithelial reticular cell framework.
- Tingible body macrophages phagocytize lymphocytes which fail to mature and enter circulation.
- Thymic corpuscles of unknown function have a degenerated central cell surrounded by multiple layers of keratinized cells.
- The blood-thymus barrier which is not permeable to antibodies is comprised of the capillary wall and a sheath of endothelial reticular cell processes.

The thymus is a primary lymphoid organ which is located in the neck and extends into the thorax within the cranial mediastinum. Epithelial cells instead of connective tissue form the framework of this organ which is seeded with developing lymphocytes from the bone marrow. The organ is comprised of lobes covered by a connective tissue capsule. The capsule extends into the lobes as septa that further divide the parenchyma into lobules. Each lobule has a cortical and a medullary region. Blood vessels traverse in the fine reticular connective tissue which surrounds the lobules. The thymus is most prominent in young animals and regresses later in life. The parenchyma of the involuted thymus is mostly replaced by adipose and connective tissues.

Cortex of the Thymus

Stellate **epithelial reticular cells** form the framework of the cortex. Each cell has a large, light-staining nucleus and several long cell processes. The processes branch and connect to cell processes extending from other epithelial reticular cells. At the periphery of the lobule, the epithelial reticular cells flatten and form a sheet around the margin of the lobule. These cells produce thymosin, thymulin, thymic humoral factor and thymopoietin, which are proteins that influence immunity and the maturation of lymphocytes.

Thymocytes (maturing T lymphocytes) occupy the space between the epithelial reticular cells. Blast thymocytes migrate from the bone marrow via the blood and locate in the periphery of the cortex where the cells undergo mitotic division. As the thymocytes continue to mature, they move from the outer thymic cortex toward the medulla. Most of the thymic lymphocytes undergo apoptosis within the cortex. Only about 1-3% are actually released into the lumen of medullary blood vessels for circulation.

Phagocytic cells called **tingible body macrophages** are interspersed among the lymphocytes. These large macrophages have remnants of apoptotic cells in their cytoplasm. Their function is to remove spent lymphocytes.

Medulla of the Thymus

Medullary epithelial reticular cells, which are somewhat larger than their cortical counterparts, form the framework in the medulla of the thymus. The medulla is lighter staining than the cortex, as fewer small lymphocytes and macrophages fill the space of the framework.

Unique **thymic corpuscles** (Hassall's corpuscles) of unknown function are also located in the medulla. The corpuscles are comprised of a central cell which has degenerated and is surrounded by layers of keratinized cells. The corpuscle may also be calcified.

Blood-Thymus Barrier

Blood vessels course in the organ capsule and enter the thymus via the connective tissue septa. The corticomedullary blood vessels then branch into the cortex as continuous capillaries. The relatively impermeable cortical capillaries are further surrounded by a sheath of epithelial reticular cell processes. Collectively, the cell processes, basement membranes, a small amount of connective tissue and the capillary endothelium form the **blood-thymus barrier.** The barrier prevents antigens from passing out of the blood and affecting nearby maturing lymphocytes within the cortex of the thymus. Cortical capillaries then empty into postcapillary venules at the corticomedullary junction.

The medulla also has a capillary bed which arises from the corticomedullary arterioles. After looping through the medulla, the medullary capillaries also terminate in the postcapillary venules. In contrast to the relatively impermeable capillaries of the cortex, the capillaries of the medulla are fenestrated.

The wall of the postcapillary venules is also highly permeable and allows lymphocytes from the thymus to enter blood circulation at this point.

Lymphatics in the thymus are primarily located in the connective tissue septa surrounding lobules, however small lymphatics have been reported in the medulla of some species.

Function of the Thymus

The thymus is seeded with stem cells from the bone marrow which proliferate in the cortex and later become immunocompetent T lymphocytes. T cells are considered mature when they express receptors that bind to self major histocompatibility complex (MHC). Lymphocytes which either bind too strongly to MHC or fail to recognize the MHC proteins undergo apoptosis. The tingible body macrophages remove the dead cells. T cells which survive the selection process then migrate into the medulla of the thymus as naive T cells. From the medulla, the T cells subsequently pass to secondary lymphoid organs such as lymph nodes and the spleen where the cells will be exposed to antigens.

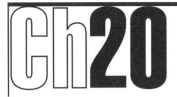

Lymph Nodes

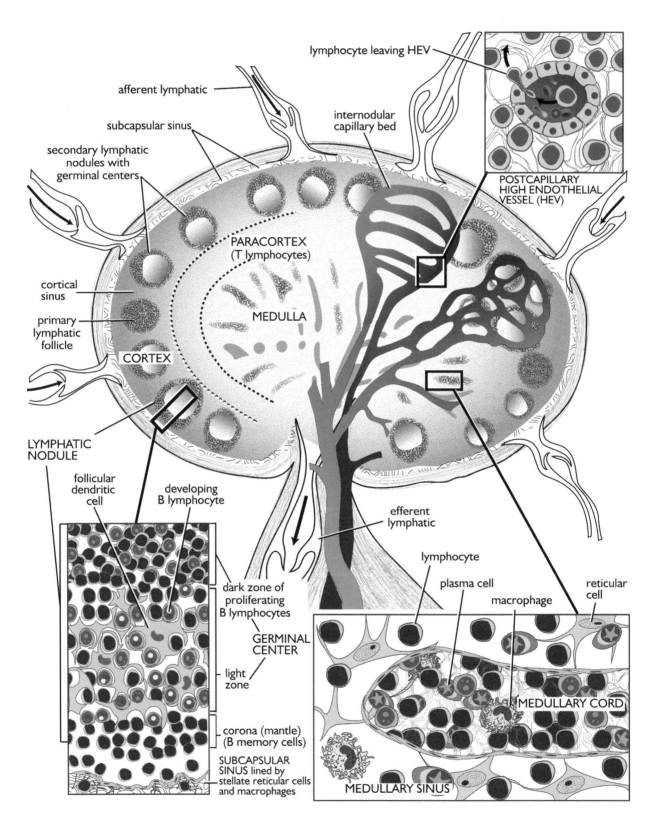

lymphocyte leaving HEV

afferent lymphatic

subcapsular sinus

internodular capillary bed

secondary lymphatic nodules with germinal centers

POSTCAPILLARY HIGH ENDOTHELIAL VESSEL (HEV)

PARACORTEX (T lymphocytes)

cortical sinus

MEDULLA

primary lymphatic follicle

CORTEX

LYMPHATIC NODULE

follicular dendritic cell

developing B lymphocyte

efferent lymphatic

lymphocyte

plasma cell

macrophage

reticular cell

dark zone of proliferating B lymphocytes

GERMINAL CENTER

light zone

MEDULLARY CORD

corona (mantle) (B memory cells)

SUBCAPSULAR SINUS lined by stellate reticular cells and macrophages

MEDULLARY SINUS

Overview

- Lymph nodes filter lymph and produce lymphocytes.
- Lymphatic nodules, cortical and medullary sinuses and medullary cords are the structural elements of the lymph node.
- Lymphatics enter along the capsule of the node and exit at the hilum.
- The germinal center of a lymphatic nodule is comprised of maturing B lymphocytes surrounded by supporting follicular dendritic cells.
- Lymph node sinuses are lined by endothelial-like reticular cells and spanned by stellate reticular cells.
- T cells are primarily located outside the follicles in the paracortical region.
- Medullary cords contain plasma cells, macrophages and reticular cells.
- Lymphocytes enter hemal nodes via the blood.
- Hemal lymph nodes filter both blood and lymph in the same sinus.

Lymph nodes are widely scattered throughout the body. Lymph, which flows in from body tissues and organs, is filtered by the node. Lymphocyte production and antigen presentation and recognition also occur in the node.

Lymph nodes contain multiple **lymphatic nodules** which are aggregates of lymphocytes. Macrophages, reticular cells, follicular dendritic cells and other dendritic cells (intraepidemal macrophages, blood dendritic cells and interdigitating cells) are also found in the node. Reticular fibers, produced by reticular cells, form the framework of the node and create a filtering meshwork in the sinuses.

Lymph Node Capsule, the Path of Lymph Flow, and Sinuses

A dense irregular connective tissue capsule surrounds the lymph node. In most species, multiple afferent lymphatics enter the node at sites along the capsule and release lymph into the **subcapsular sinus** immediately beneath the capsule. From the subcapsular sinus, the lymph continues through **cortical sinuses** and then **medullary sinuses.** Efferent lymph leaves the node through lymphatics at the hilum.

The sinuses of the lymph node are lined by endothelial-like reticular cells. Stellate reticular cells and reticular fibers span the sinus lumen and slow the flow of lymph, allowing for more interaction between lymphocytes and antigens in the node. Macrophages are also attached to the reticular cell framework.

Cortex of the Lymph Node

The lymph node cortex has multiple lymphatic nodules separated by cortical sinuses. Active lymphatic nodules have a light-staining **germinal center** that contains large, euchromatic B lymphocytes and surrounding follicular dendritic cells. Lymphocytes in the germinal center are capable of active proliferation. **Follicular dendritic cells** support the B cells and are thought to assemble the cells into follicles. The germinal center is surrounded by a dark-staining **corona** (mantle) comprised of small lymphocytes in the process of migrating from the germinal center. T cells are primarily located outside the follicles in the paracortex.

During maturation, B cells are exposed to antigens by antigen-presenting cells. The B cells then express surface immunoglobulins and become either B memory cells or plasma cells which then leave the nodule.

Cortical sinuses extend between the nodules from the subcapsular sinus to the medulla. The cortical sinuses are continuous with medullary sinuses.

Paracortex of the Lymph Node

The **paracortex** (inner cortex) is located at the junction between the cortex and medulla, and represents a site of T cell maturation. Few lymphatic nodules are present. Other cells in the paracortical region include reticular cells and interdigitating cells. **Interdigitating cells** migrate into the paracortex from other regions of the body and present their antigens to T cells. The activated T cells then move to the medullary sinuses and exit the node.

Medulla of the Lymph Node

The medulla of the lymph node is less cellular than the cortex and therefore stains lighter. Lymphatic nodules are lacking in the medulla in most species except the pig, which has nodules in the medulla but lacks them in the cortex.

The medullary region of the node is arranged in cellular **medullary cords** which are located between **medullary sinuses.** Cells of the cords include B memory and T lymphocytes, plasma cells, macrophages, and reticular cells which form the framework of the cords along with reticular fibers. Lymph in the medullary sinuses empties into the subcapsular sinus at the hilus and then into an efferent lymph vessel leaving the node.

Blood Supply of the Lymph Node

Blood vessels enter the node at the hilum and travel through the connective tissue into the medullary cords, reducing in size to form capillary beds. The medullary capillaries extend into the cortex and eventually form unique postcapillary venules called **high endothelial vessels** (HEVs). These vessels are lined by tall simple cuboidal endothelium and represent a point of exit for lymphocytes recirculating from the blood into the node. HEVs drain into larger veins which exit the node at the hilum.

Hemal Nodes and Hemal Lymph Nodes

Hemal nodes, found primarily in ruminants, lack lymphatics. For the maturation phase of development, lymphocytes enter and exit the hemal node via the blood.

Hemal lymph nodes, which have characteristics of both the lymph node and hemal node, are present in the sheep and goat.

Lymphatic Vessels

Lymphatic vessels conduct lymph from various regions of the body to the lymph nodes. Lymphatics are lined by endothelium surrounded by a thin layer of connective tissue. Valves are usually present in lymphatics.

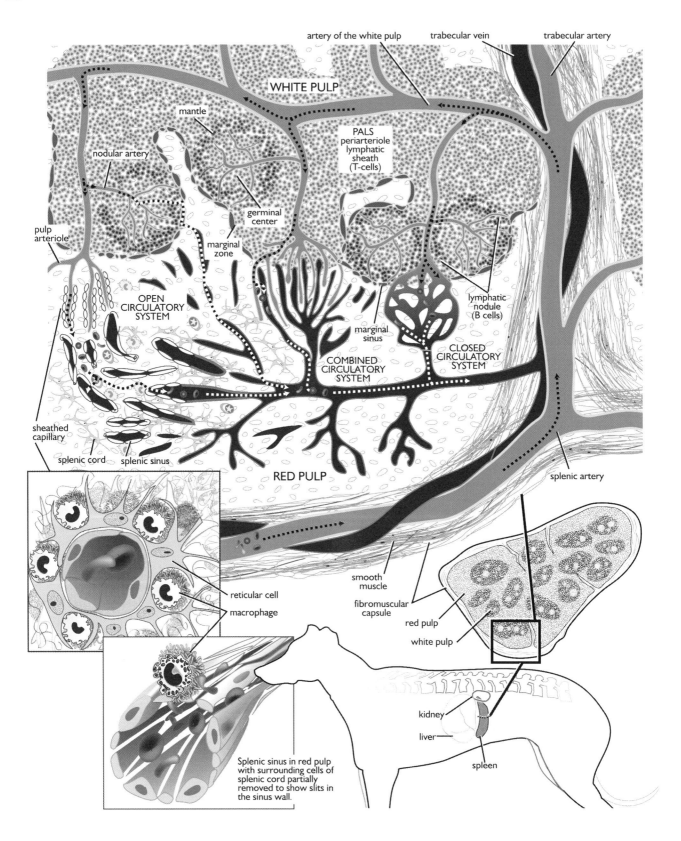

artery of the white pulp

trabecular vein

trabecular artery

WHITE PULP

mantle

nodular artery

PALS
periarteriole
lymphatic
sheath
(T-cells)

germinal
center

pulp
arteriole

marginal
zone

OPEN
CIRCULATORY
SYSTEM

lymphatic
nodule
(B cells)

marginal
sinus

COMBINED
CIRCULATORY
SYSTEM

CLOSED
CIRCULATORY
SYSTEM

sheathed
capillary

splenic cord

splenic sinus

RED PULP

splenic artery

reticular cell

macrophage

smooth
muscle

fibromuscular
capsule

red pulp

white pulp

kidney

liver

spleen

Splenic sinus in red pulp
with surrounding cells of
splenic cord partially
removed to show slits in
the sinus wall.

Overview

- The spleen has both red pulp consisting of splenic cords and blood-filled sinuses and white pulp containing large numbers of lymphocytes.
- The white pulp forms periarteriolar lymphatic sheaths and lymphatic nodules around blood vessels entering the spleen.
- T lymphocytes predominate in the PALS while B lymphocytes predominate in nodules.
- In closed circulation through the spleen, blood empties from the vessels of the white pulp into sheathed capillaries of the red pulp and then directly into the sinuses.
- In open circulation, blood empties from the sheathed capillaries into the splenic cords and then enters the sinuses through slits in the wall.

The spleen filters and stores blood, participates in blood cell formation in the fetus, and removes spent erythrocytes. An immune response against blood-borne antigens is also mounted by the spleen.

Lymphatic nodules are scattered throughout the parenchyma of the spleen. A defined cortex and medulla found in other organs of the immune system is not present. Instead, the spleen is organized as **red pulp,** consisting of blood-filled sinuses and cords of splenic cells, or **white pulp,** containing large numbers of lymphocytes. White pulp is abundant in a so-called defensive spleen while red pulp predominates in a storage spleen.

Capsule of the Spleen

The spleen is surrounded by a connective tissue capsule with variable amounts of smooth muscle, depending on the species. Smooth muscle may relax when barbiturate anesthesia is administered, causing the capsule to expand and allowing the spleen to engorge with blood. The capsule can also contract, forcing stored blood into peripheral circulation. Connective tissue trabeculae extend from the capsule into the parenchyma.

White Pulp of the Spleen

The white pulp is comprised of **periarteriolor lymphatic sheaths** (PALS) and **lymphatic nodules** with associated efferent lymphatics. Large numbers of lymphocytes account for the basophilic staining. Reticular cells and reticular fibers form the supporting network for the white pulp.

PALS are sheaths of cells which surround arteries passing into the parenchyma from the connective tissue trabeculae. Adjacent to the tunica media of the vessel, T lymphocytes predominate. In the periphery of the sheath, both T and B lymphocytes, macrophages and dendritic cells are present.

Lymphatic nodules of the spleen are scattered along the blood vessels within the white pulp and may or may not have active germinal centers. B lymphocytes predominate in the nodules.

Red Pulp of the Spleen

Splenic sinuses and cellular splenic cords form the red pulp. The sinuses are lined by longitudinal endothelial cells which can contract and allow gaps to form between the cells. Reticular fibers surround the fenestrated basement membrane of the endothelium and create supporting structure for the sinus wall.

Splenic cords form a network around the outside of the sinuses. The cords contain erythrocytes, macrophages, plasma cells and lymphocytes within a framework of reticular cells and fibers.

Marginal Zone of the Spleen

The marginal zone is located between the red and white pulp. Reticular cells surround the periphery of the white pulp and extend into the red pulp. Capillaries from the white pulp drain into venous sinuses of the red pulp at the marginal zone. Slow-flowing blood in the sinuses can then contact local macrophages and lymphocytes, and initiate an immune response.

Blood Supply to the Spleen

Blood flows into the spleen via the splenic artery which then branches into trabecular arteries. As an individual **trabecular artery** emerges from the connective tissue, it is then known as the **artery of the white pulp** (central artery) which is surrounded by the PALS. The blood vessel continues into a lymphatic nodule as the **nodular artery.** The nodular artery becomes smaller and terminates in the marginal zone or forms a vascular tuft (penicillus) in the red pulp.

Blood vessels from the white pulp, known as **pulp arterioles,** continue in the red pulp as **sheathed capillaries.** The sheathed capillaries are surrounded by macrophages and a network of reticular cells and fibers.

Two theories predominate relative to the connection between the sheathed capillaries and the venous circulation. The **closed circulation theory** proposes that blood empties from the capillary directly into the splenic sinus. In the **open circulation theory,** blood empties into spaces between the reticular cells of the red pulp outside the sinus and then enters circulation through slits in the sinus wall. Another theory says that the methods of circulation alternate between closed and open based on physiologic need.

Blood then continues through the terminal sinuses or venule to exit the spleen through the trabecular vein.

Blood Filtration Mechanisms in the Spleen

As blood passes through splenic sinuses, the endothelium of the sinuses traps defective erythrocytes and prevents their reentry into the blood. This process is termed **mechanical filtration.**

Biological filtration occurs as macrophages recognize non-functional blood cells and remove them from the splenic circulation.

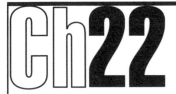

Mucosa-Associated Lymphatic Tissue

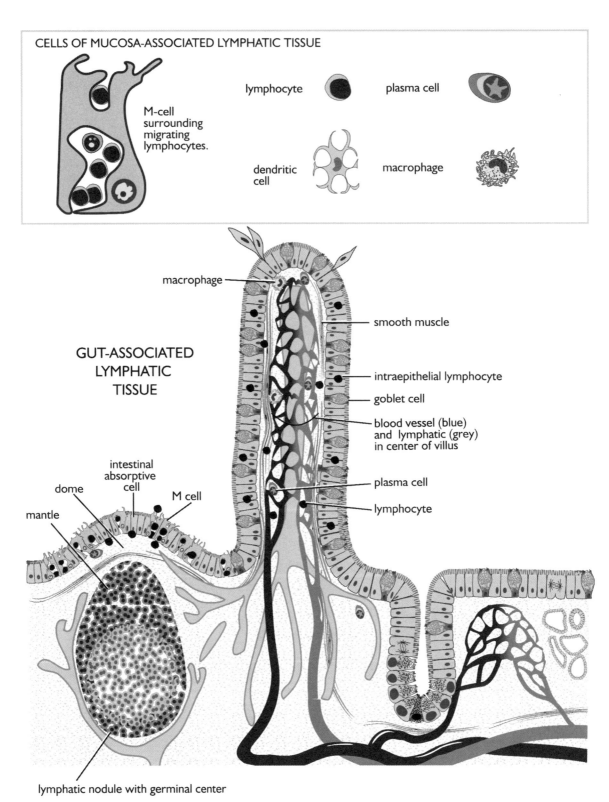

CELLS OF MUCOSA-ASSOCIATED LYMPHATIC TISSUE

M-cell surrounding migrating lymphocytes.

lymphocyte

plasma cell

dendritic cell

macrophage

GUT-ASSOCIATED LYMPHATIC TISSUE

macrophage

smooth muscle

intraepithelial lymphocyte

goblet cell

blood vessel (blue) and lymphatic (grey) in center of villus

plasma cell

lymphocyte

dome

intestinal absorptive cell

M cell

mantle

lymphatic nodule with germinal center

Overview

- Solitary and aggregated lymphatic nodules are associated with most mucous membranes and are known as MALT.
- Groups of MALT associated with the gut and respiratory system are referred to as GALT and BALT respectively.
- Mucosal lymphatic nodules have epithelial M cells, dome area cells, and B and T lymphocytes.
- Diffuse lymphatic tissue lies within the lamina epithelialis or the lamina propria.
- Tonsils are encapsulated lymphatic nodules that are located in the oropharynx and nasopharynx.
- The cloacal bursa in avians is the site B cell maturation.

Lymphatic tissue is distributed in many other locations throughout the body besides the lymph nodes, spleen and thymus. Diffuse and nodular lymphoid tissue serves as a line of host defense. Lymphoid tissue located under mucous membranes is referred to in general terms as **mucosa-associated lymphatic tissue** (MALT). Specific groups of MALT nodules include **gut-associated lymphatic tissue** (GALT) of the digestive system, **bronchiolar-associated lymphatic tissue** (BALT) of the respiratory system, **tonsils** and the **cloacal bursa** of birds. Mucosal lymphatic tissues receive antigens and secrete antibodies via the overlying surface epithelium rather than through the lymphatic or blood circulations.

Diffuse Mucosal Lymphatic Tissue

Throughout the mucosa, populations of lymphocytes are found within the epithelium or the lamina propria. **Intraepithelial lymphocytes** are numerous and represent a unique population of T cells which express CD8 surface proteins. Expression of CD8 indicates that these cells have the ability to kill cells that have foreign molecules on their surfaces. CD8 lymphocytes develop from bone marrow rather than thymic populations of lymphocytes. Beyond production of cytokines, the function of intraepithelial lymphocytes is poorly understood.

Immune cells in the lamina propria include T and B cells, macrophages, dendritic and mast cells. T lymphocytes in the lamina propria primarily express CD4 surface proteins and are recognized as helper cells which promote proliferation, development and immune function of other cells. B cells in the lamina propria are mostly plasma cells which produce antibodies. Dendritic cells act as antigen-presenting cells while macrophages in the lamina propria are primarily phagocytic.

Gut-Associated Lymphatic Tissue (GALT)

Solitary and aggregated lymphatic nodules are located along the length of the digestive tract. In the small intestine, aggregated lymphatic nodules (Peyer's patches) may elevate the overlying intestinal epithelium and are most numerous in the ileum.

The epithelium over the lymphatic nodules contains **M cells** (microfold cells) which are located among other intestinal absorptive cells. The M cells have poorly developed microvilli when compared to absorptive cells. The basement membrane beneath the M cell is discontinuous and allows lymphocytes to migrate and localize in invaginations of the basal membrane of the cell. Foreign materials on the epithelial surface, such as bacteria, are pinocytosed by the M cells, and antigens are presented to the underlying cells. Goblet cells are lacking in the epithelium over the nodule where M cells are present.

Dome area cells, a dense region of dendritic cells immediately beneath the epithelium, receive antigens emerging from the M cells. These cells present the antigens to underlying T cells.

Follicular **B and T lymphocytes** comprise the rest of the lymphatic nodules.

Bronchiolar-Associated Lymphatic Tissue (BALT)

Lymphatic nodules are also found in the walls of the bronchi and bronchioles. These nodules are similar to the GALT.

Tonsils

Palatine tonsils are located at the junction of the oral cavity and oropharynx. The epithelium of the palatine tonsil in horses, ruminants and swine has deep invaginations called **crypts** which extend into the underlying lymphatic tissue. The lingual tonsil is located in the base of the tongue and the pharyngeal tonsil is found in the wall of the nasopharynx. Lymphatic nodules are usually surrounded by a capsule.

Cloacal Bursa in Avians

Most birds do not have lymph nodes. The function of mammalian nodes is taken over by diffuse lymphatic tissues and a lymphatic organ in the dorsal wall of the cloaca called the **cloacal bursa** (bursa of Fabricus).

B cell precursors migrate to the bursa early in development and lymphopoiesis occurs in the folds of the organ. Surface epithelium of the bursa has the ability to present antigen to the underlying developing lymphocytes, thus stimulating production of a diverse population of immunocompetent lymphocytes.

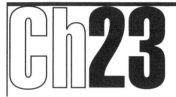
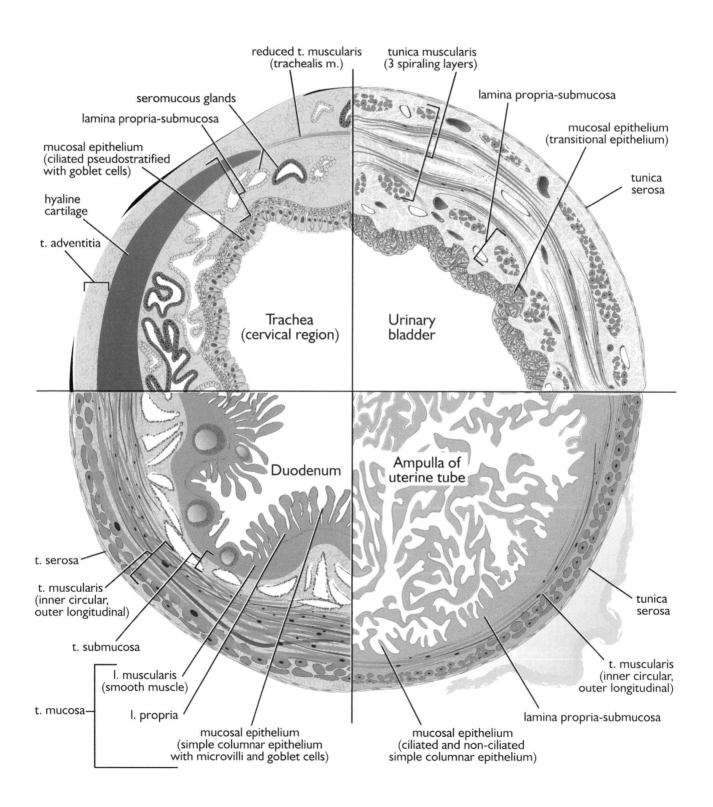

reduced t. muscularis
(trachealis m.)

tunica muscularis
(3 spiraling layers)

seromucous glands

lamina propria-submucosa

lamina propria-submucosa

mucosal epithelium
(ciliated pseudostratified
with goblet cells)

mucosal epithelium
(transitional epithelium)

tunica
serosa

hyaline
cartilage

t. adventitia

Trachea
(cervical region)

Urinary
bladder

Duodenum

Ampulla of
uterine tube

t. serosa

t. muscularis
(inner circular,
outer longitudinal)

t. submucosa

tunica
serosa

l. muscularis
(smooth muscle)

t. muscularis
(inner circular,
outer longitudinal)

t. mucosa

l. propria

lamina propria-submucosa

mucosal epithelium
(simple columnar epithelium
with microvilli and goblet cells)

mucosal epithelium
(ciliated and non-ciliated
simple columnar epithelium)

Overview

- The tunica mucosa is comprised of mucosal epithelium, a lamina propria of connective tissue and a lamina muscularis of smooth muscle.
- The tela submucosa is connective tissue which often blends with the lamina propria if the lamina muscularis is absent.
- Layers of smooth muscle form the tunica muscularis.
- The outer surface of the organ is covered with connective tissue called the tunica adventitia, or mesothelium and a small amount of underlying connective tissue which forms the tunica serosa.

The wall of tubular organs has several named layers or tunics. These layers vary from organ to organ so a basic pattern will be presented here and variations will be discussed with individual organs.

Tunica Mucosa

The tunica mucosa includes mucosal epithelium, lamina propria and lamina muscularis. **Mucosal epithelium** (lamina epithelialis) lines the lumen of the tubular organ and varies in structure. A layer of mucus produced by the epithelium or associated glands covers the epithelial surface.

The **lamina propria** lies beneath the basement membrane complex of the mucosal epithelium and is composed of areolar connective tissue. Glands and lymphatic tissue may also be present in the lamina propria.

A thin layer of smooth muscle forms the **lamina muscularis** which is absent in many organs. When the lamina muscularis is not present, the connective tissue of the lamina propria and the connective tissue of the underlying submucosa blend into a propria-submucosa with no clear separation between the layers. The muscularis layer facilitates contractile movements of the mucosa, and release of secretions from glands in the lamina propria.

Tela Submucosa

The tela submucosa lies deep to the tunica mucosa. The connective tissue of this layer has a web like appearance and thus the layer is referred to as a tela rather than a tunic. Glands and other structures such as the cartilage rings of the trachea and submucosal ganglia may also be present in this layer.

Tunica Muscularis

Two or more layers of smooth muscle form the tunica muscularis. When two layers are present, the inner layer of muscle cells is generally oriented in a circular fashion around the organ while cells in the outer layer run longitudinally. Vascular and neural plexi are often present between the muscle layers.

Tunica Adventitia or Tunica Serosa

The outermost layer of a tubular organ is either a tunica adventitia or a tunica serosa. The tunica adventitia is connective tissue which blends with connective tissue of adjacent organs or structures. Mesothelial cells and a small amount of underlying connective tissue form the tunica serosa which is present when organs are adjacent to a body cavity.

The tunica serosa of the heart is the pericardium. On the surface of the lungs adjacent to the pleural cavity, the serosa is the visceral pleura. The visceral peritoneum is the serosal layer of the abdominal viscera.

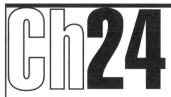

Respiratory System

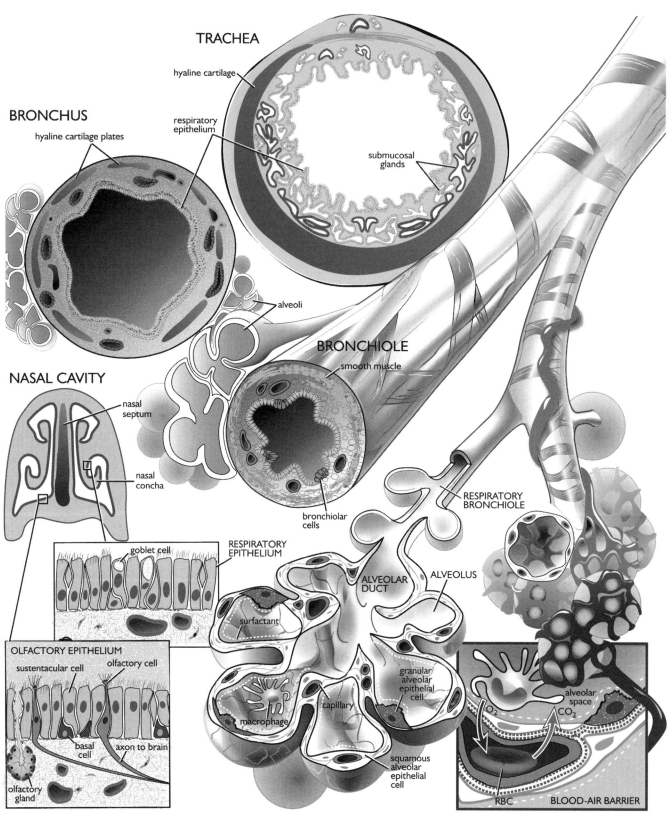

TRACHEA

hyaline cartilage

respiratory epithelium

submucosal glands

BRONCHUS

hyaline cartilage plates

alveoli

BRONCHIOLE

smooth muscle

NASAL CAVITY

nasal septum

nasal concha

bronchiolar cells

RESPIRATORY BRONCHIOLE

RESPIRATORY EPITHELIUM

goblet cell

ALVEOLAR DUCT

ALVEOLUS

surfactant

granular alveolar epithelial cell

OLFACTORY EPITHELIUM

sustentacular cell

olfactory cell

capillary

macrophage

O_2

CO_2

alveolar space

basal cell

axon to brain

squamous alveolar epithelial cell

olfactory gland

RBC

BLOOD-AIR BARRIER

Overview

- Respiratory and olfactory epithelia line the nasal cavity and cover the nasal conchae.
- Olfactory cells are bipolar neurons which participate in the sense of smell.
- The supporting structure of the larynx is comprised of elastic and hyaline cartilage
- C-shaped hyaline cartilage rings support the wall of the trachea which is lined with respiratory epithelium.
- Bronchi are characterized by hyaline cartilage plates in the propria-submucosa.
- Bronchioles lack cartilage and have extensive smooth muscle in their walls.
- Gas exchange occurs across alveolar epithelial cells while granular alveolar cells produce surfactant.

The respiratory system conducts air from the nasal cavity to the lungs where gas exchange occurs.

External Nose

The external surface of the nose is covered with keratinized stratified squamous epithelium with characteristic grooves. Varying amounts of pigment are present in the epithelial cells. The shape of the nose is determined by internal hyaline cartilage.

Nasal Cavity

Lining epithelium of the nasal cavity is ciliated pseudostratified columnar epithelium with goblet cells, also known as **respiratory epithelium.** Secretions from mixed serous and mucous glands humidify the incoming air, while submucosal vascular tissue provides thermoregulation.

The nasal cavity is divided on the midline by the cartilaginous **nasal septum.** Deeper in the nasal cavity, bony scrolls called **nasal conchae** extend off the lateral wall. The conchae are covered by respiratory epithelium and specialized regions of **olfactory epithelium.**

Olfactory epithelium is comprised of sustentacular, basal and olfactory cells. The uppermost layer of epithelial nuclei belong to supportive **sustentacular cells** which are columnar shaped and have surface microvilli. The nuclei of epithelial stem cells, the **basal cells,** form the deepest nuclear layer. The balance of the nuclei belong to **olfactory cells** which are bipolar neurons with non-motile cilia. Soluble components of odors are taken up by the olfactory cell. Chemical reaction then generates electrical impulses which are sent to the brain via axons of the olfactory nerve. Olfaction is assisted by serous secretions from **olfactory glands** (Bowman's glands) beneath the olfactory epithelium.

Vomeronasal Organ

The vomeronasal organ is a paired, tubular structure in the floor of the nasal cavity. The lateral surface of the tubule is lined with respiratory epithelium while the medial surface is lined with olfactory epithelium. The vomeronasal organ plays a role in chemoreception of soluble compounds.

Nasopharynx

The nasopharynx connects the nasal cavity to the pharynx. Respiratory epithelium lines the cavity and both diffuse and aggregated lymphatic tissues are present beneath the epithelium. The pharyngeal tonsil is located in the roof of the nasopharynx.

Larynx

The larynx connects the pharynx to the trachea. Stratified squamous epithelium lines the larynx and transitions to respiratory epithelium before reaching the trachea. Elastic cartilage forms the epiglottis and corniculate process of the arytenoid cartilage. The remaining laryngeal cartilages are comprised of hyaline cartilage. Lymphatic tissue is present between the epithelium and the cartilage.

Trachea

The trachea is lined by respiratory epithelium. Seromucous submucosal glands produce tracheal secretions which are swept toward the larynx by the epithelial cilia. C-shaped hyaline cartilage rings in the propria-submucosa provide shape and support for the tracheal wall. Smooth muscle connects the ends of the tracheal ring. The trachea is surrounded by a tunica adventitia.

Lung

Just before entering the lung, the trachea branches into individual **bronchi.** Each bronchus is lined with respiratory epithelium. Hyaline cartilage in the propria-submucosa is arranged in multiple plates.

Bronchi branch to smaller **bronchioles** and the lining epithelium decreases in height to simple cuboidal epithelium. In this region, the epithelium is comprised of **bronchiolar cells** (Clara cells), ciliated lining cells, and neuroendocrine cells. Dome-shaped bronchiolar cells have microvilli and are thought to produce protective glycoproteins and metabolize toxins. The cartilage present in upper airways is replaced by prominent smooth muscle.

Bronchioles continue as **respiratory bronchioles.** Gas exchange occurs in the alveoli which protrude from the walls of the respiratory bronchiole.

The **alveolar duct** connects the respiratory bronchiole with the **alveolar sac,** a cluster of alveoli. Smooth muscle is diminished to small patches in the wall of the duct.

The **alveolus** is a thin-walled structure where gas exchange occurs in the lung. Squamous **alveolar epithelial cells** are the primary lining cell. Scattered **granular alveolar epithelial cells** produce surfactant which maintains surface tension in the alveolus. In the lumen, **alveolar macrophages** remove particulate material from the epithelial surface.

Blood-Air Barrier

The pulmonary artery forms an extensive capillary bed within the lung. Gas exchange occurs across the **blood-air barrier,** consisting of the squamous alveolar epithelial cell, basement membrane of the epithelium, the septal space containing connective tissue and cells, the basement membrane of the pulmonary capillary and the capillary endothelial cell.

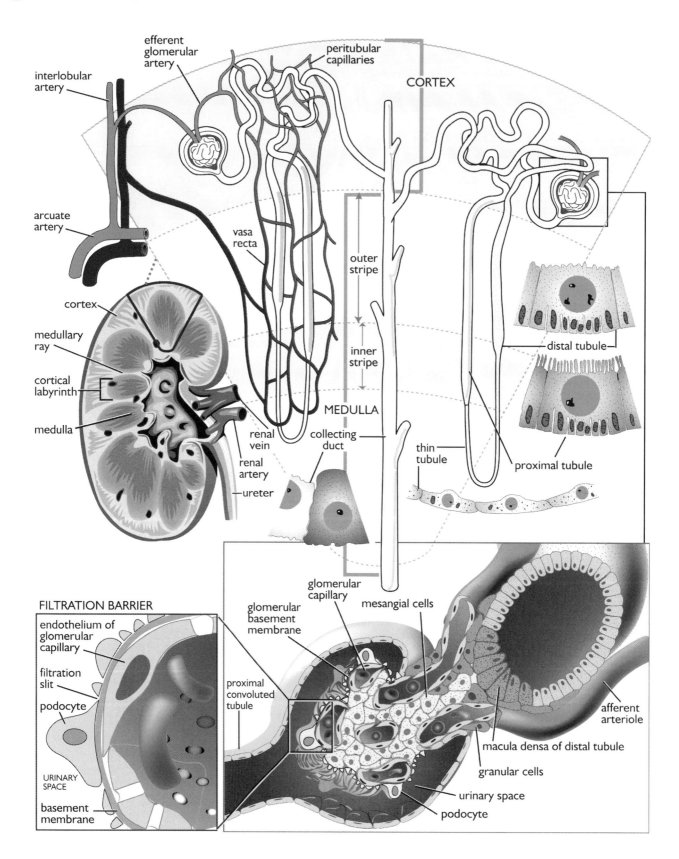

efferent glomerular artery

peritubular capillaries

CORTEX

interlobular artery

arcuate artery

vasa recta

outer stripe

inner stripe

cortex

medullary ray

cortical labyrinth

medulla

MEDULLA

renal vein

renal artery

ureter

collecting duct

thin tubule

distal tubule

proximal tubule

FILTRATION BARRIER

endothelium of glomerular capillary

filtration slit

podocyte

URINARY SPACE

basement membrane

glomerular capillary

glomerular basement membrane

mesangial cells

proximal convoluted tubule

afferent arteriole

macula densa of distal tubule

granular cells

urinary space

podocyte

Overview

- The nephron includes a renal corpuscle, proximal convoluted and straight tubules, thin tubule, distal straight and convoluted tubules, and collecting duct.
- A glomerular capillary and surrounding glomerular capsule form the renal corpuscle.
- Urine components cross the filtration barrier which includes the glomerular endothelium, basement membrane and the filtration slit between podocytes.
- The proximal and distal tubules and collecting ducts are lined with variable simple cuboidal epithelium.
- The macula densa, mesangial cells and granular cells form the juxtaglomerular apparatus.

The kidneys filter blood, reabsorb water and electrolytes, and eliminate metabolic wastes as urine. In addition, hormones such as erythropoietin, renin and angiotensin II are produced by the kidneys.

Renal Cortex

The cortex of a kidney contains the **cortical labyrinth** and **medullary rays.** The cortical labyrinth includes the renal corpuscles and both distal and proximal convoluted tubules. Medullary rays are comprised of the straight tubules and collecting ducts.

Renal Medulla

The outer medulla of the kidney contains straight tubules and collecting ducts in the outer stripe and straight tubules, collecting ducts and thin tubules in the inner stripe. Thin tubules and collecting ducts are located in the inner medulla.

Nephron

The nephron is the structural and functional unit of the kidney. Each nephron includes a renal corpuscle, proximal convoluted and straight tubules, thin tubule, distal straight and convoluted tubules and a collecting duct.

Renal Corpuscle

The **renal glomerulus,** a convoluted capillary tuft, forms the central structure of the renal corpuscle. The porous capillary is surrounded by the **glomerular basement membrane. Mesangial cells** outside the capillary provide support.

The renal glomerulus is surrounded by a **glomerular capsule** (Bowman's capsule) comprised of two layers. The visceral layer is formed by **podocytes** which envelope the glomerular capillary. Extensive cell processes branch and are termed **pedicels** at the tertiary level. Between the pedicels, the **filtration slit** is filled with an electron-dense layer called the **slit diaphragm.** Simple squamous epithelium forms the parietal layer of the glomerular capsule. The space between the two layers of the capsule is termed the **urinary space.**

An ultrafiltrate of blood crosses the **filtration barrier** to form urine in the urinary space. The barrier includes the glomerular capillary endothelium, basement membrane, and the slit diaphragm between the podocytes.

Proximal Tubule

The urinary space of the glomerular capsule empties into the proximal tubule. The initial portion of the tubule in the cortical labyrinth is more highly convoluted than the final portion which is located in the medullary rays. The **proximal tubule** is lined by simple cuboidal epithelium with a well-developed apical border of microvilli. Lateral cell junctions are leaky, allowing passive transport between cells.

Thin Tubule

The proximal tubule continues as the thin tubule which is lined by simple squamous epithelium. The epithelial nuclei of the thin tubule are spherical and protrude into the lumen more than those of nearby endothelial cells of adjacent capillaries.

Distal Tubule

The **distal tubule** continues from the thin tubule as a straight segment which begins at the junction of the inner and outer medulla, passes the pole of the renal corpuscle and ends as the convoluted segment before emptying into the collecting duct. The distal tubule is lined by simple cuboidal epithelium with few, short microvilli and tight intercellular junctions restricting transport between cells.

Collecting Duct

The final segment of the nephron, the **collecting duct,** is lined by simple cuboidal epithelium which has both light-staining **principal cells** and darker-staining **intercalated cells.** Intercalated cells change their shape to either protrude into the lumen or retract, depending on their secretory state.

Blood Supply

Blood enters the kidney through the renal artery which branches as the **interlobar artery.** The interlobar artery continues as the **arcuate artery** and then branches between lobules as **interlobular artery.** The interlobular artery give rise to an **afferent glomerular arteriole** which forms the glomerular capillary bed and then exits as the **efferent glomerular arteriole** to form a second capillary bed. Superficial and midcortical glomerular blood vessels provide a capillary network surrounding the tubules of the cortex, while juxtamedullary glomeruli form the **vasa recta** capillary bed surrounding the straight and thin tubules of the medulla (loop of Henle).

Juxtaglomerular Apparatus

The juxtaglomerular apparatus is located at the vascular pole of the renal corpuscle. The **macula densa,** a dense region of epithelial cells in the wall of the distal straight tubule, senses the composition of fluid in the distal tubule and provides feedback to cells in the wall of the afferent arteriole to control blood flow through the glomerulus. **Mesangial cells,** located between the macula densa and the afferent and efferent glomerular arterioles, are thought to be phagocytic. **Granular cells** in the tunica media of the afferent arteriole produce renin which increases reabsorption in distal tubules and constricts the afferent arteriole.

Ureter, Urinary Bladder, Urethra

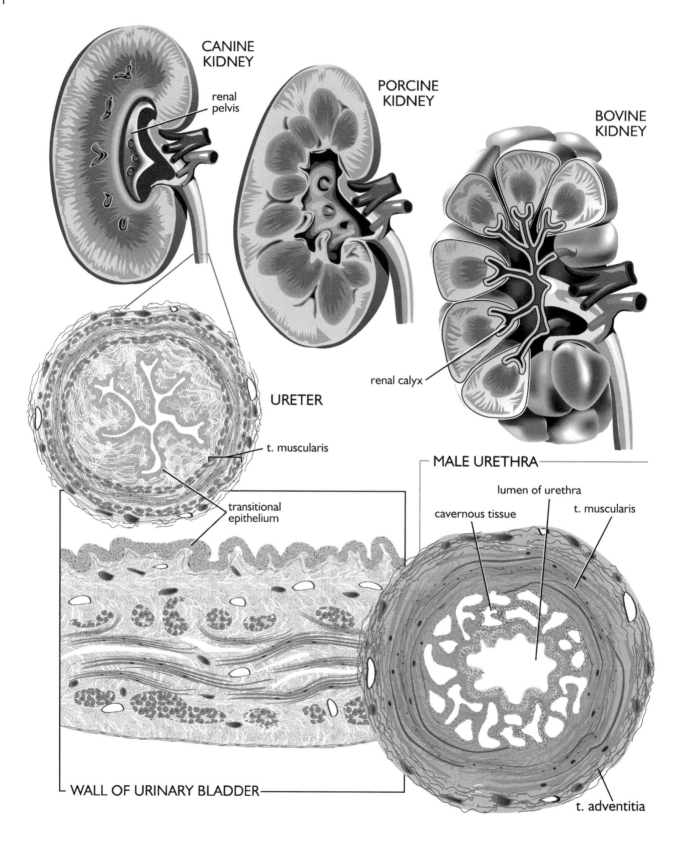

CANINE KIDNEY

renal pelvis

PORCINE KIDNEY

BOVINE KIDNEY

renal calyx

URETER

t. muscularis

transitional epithelium

MALE URETHRA

lumen of urethra

cavernous tissue

t. muscularis

WALL OF URINARY BLADDER

t. adventitia

Overview

- The urinary passages from the kidney to the cranial ureter are lined with transitional epithelium. Stratified squamous epithelium lines the distal ureter near the external opening.
- The smooth muscle of the tunica muscularis is arranged as three layers in the ureter, irregular bundles in the urinary bladder, and two to three irregular layers in the urethra.
- Cavernous vascular spaces are present in the lamina propria-submucosa of the urethra.

Urine from the collecting ducts of the nephrons enters the papillary ducts and drains from the medulla into either the renal pelvis or renal calyces. Urine is then transported through the ureter, urinary bladder and urethra. The urinary bladder serves as a temporary storage reservoir for urine until it can be eliminated from the body.

Renal Pelvis and Renal Calyces

The kidney of dogs, cats, and horses has a renal pelvis which represents the initial expanded segment of the ureter. Fusion of the medullary pyramids results in the formation of a renal crest which is more prominent in carnivores and small in the horse. Mucous glands are present in the tunica mucosa of the renal pelvis of the horse.

In cattle, the ducts of the pyramids empty into several renal calyces (cup-like structures) which converge to form the ureter. A renal pelvis is not present.

The kidney of pigs has both minor calyces and a renal pelvis which leads to the ureter.

Both the renal pelvis and renal calyces are lined by transitional epithelium.

Ureter

The ureter is a tubular structure with a narrow, stellate lumen. Transitional epithelium forms the lining layer. The lamina propria-submucosa is connective tissue proper. Three layers of smooth muscle form the tunica muscularis. The smooth muscle fibers in the inner and outer layers are arranged in a longitudinal pattern, while fibers in the middle layer are oriented circularly. Either a tunica adventitia or tunica serosa is present as the outermost layer of the ureter.

In the horse, epithelial goblet cells and numerous mucous submucosal glands are present in the ureter wall, and contribute to the mucous content of equine urine.

Urinary Bladder

The urinary bladder is lined with transitional epithelium. A lamina muscularis mucosa of smooth muscle is present in the horse, ruminant, dog and pig but is lacking in the cat. The tunica muscularis is comprised of a thick layer of smooth muscle arranged in irregular bundles. A tunica serosa surrounds the urinary bladder.

Urethra

Transitional epithelium continues from the urinary bladder as the lining of the urethra. Near the external body opening, the epithelium changes from transitional to stratified squamous. At the transition point, stratified cuboidal or stratified columnar epithelium may be present. Cavernous spaces lined with endothelium vary in number in the lamina propria-submucosa. In the spongiose portion of the male urethra, the cavernous spaces greatly increase to form the corpus spongiosum. The tunica muscularis is comprised of two to three layers of smooth muscle which are irregularly arranged. Skeletal muscle is present in the tunica muscularis at the caudal end of the urethra. The outer layer of the urethra is formed by a tunica adventitia.

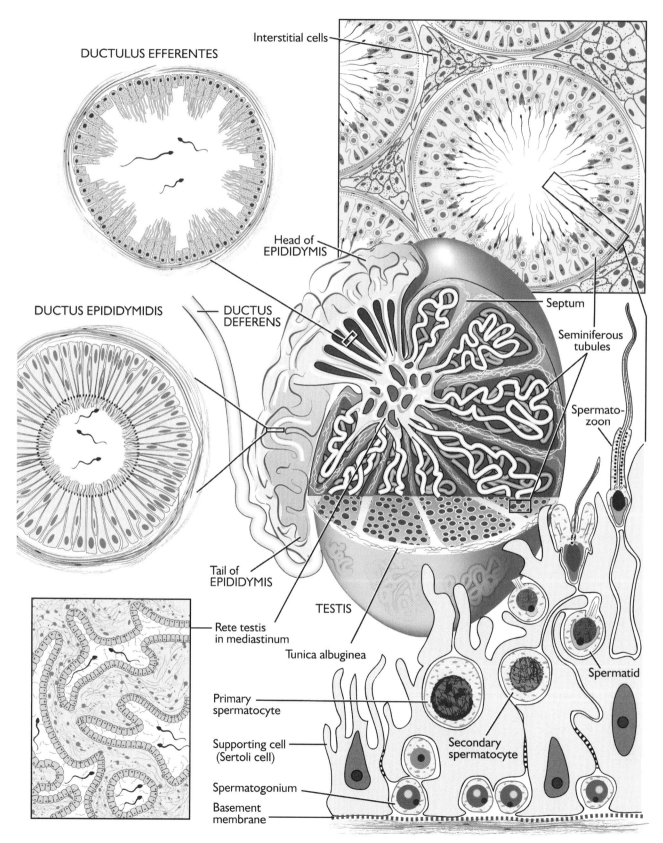

DUCTULUS EFFERENTES

DUCTUS EPIDIDYMIDIS

DUCTUS DEFERENS

Interstitial cells

Head of EPIDIDYMIS

Septum

Seminiferous tubules

Spermato-zoon

Tail of EPIDIDYMIS

TESTIS

Rete testis in mediastinum

Tunica albuginea

Spermatid

Primary spermatocyte

Secondary spermatocyte

Supporting cell (Sertoli cell)

Spermatogonium

Basement membrane

Overview

- Supporting and spermatogenic cells form the epithelium of the convoluted seminiferous tubules.
- The spermatogonium, primary spermatocyte, secondary spermatocyte, spermatid and spermatozoa represent the stages of sperm development.
- The ductuli efferentes is lined by ciliated and non-ciliated epithelial cells while the ductus epididymis is lined by pseudostratified epithelium with stereocilia.
- Accessory glands are characterized by epithelial infoldings in the vesicular gland, mucous epithelium in the bulbourethral gland and pseudostratified epithelium in the prostate.
- The male urethra is surrounded by cavernous erectile tissue within the penis.

The male reproductive system includes the testis, epididymis, ductus deferens and accessory glands. These structures produce semen consisting of spermatozoa and associated secretions.

Testis

In the testis, spermatozoa are produced for exocrine secretion, as well as hormones for endocrine secretion.

The epithelium of the **convoluted seminiferous tubules** includes supporting cells and spermatogenic cells. The **supporting cells** (Sertoli cells), located in the basal region of the epithelium, surround the adjacent spermatogenic cells. Tightly bound to other supporting cells, they create a **blood-testis barrier** which shields the developing spermatogenic cells from blood-borne influence. **Spermatogenic cells** in various stages of development comprise the balance of the cell population. The basally-located **spermatogonium** is capable of mitosis. The largest cell, the **primary spermatocyte,** undergoes the first meiotic division while the **secondary spermatocyte** completes the second meiotic division. The resulting **spermatid** is haploid and becomes the **spermatozoon** which represents the final developmental stage.

Clusters of endocrine **interstitial cells** (Leydig cells) are located between the convoluted seminiferous tubules. Interstitial cells produce testosterone.

Straight seminiferous tubules, lined by simple cuboidal epithelium, connect the convoluted tubules to the rete testis. The **rete testis** consists of irregular anastomosing channels which lead to the ductuli efferentes of the epididymis.

Epididymis

As the spermatozoa pass through the epididymis, they become motile and surface receptors are activated.

Simple columnar epithelial cells line the **ductuli efferentes** of the epididymis. Ciliated cells help propel spermatozoa along the tubules while the microvilli on non-ciliated cells are important in fluid reabsorption. Smooth muscle cells increase in the wall of the distal ductuli efferentes.

The **ductus epididymidis,** lined by pseudostratified columnar epithelium with stereocilia, continues from the efferent ductules.

Ductus Deferens

The ductus deferens, located in the spermatic cord, is a continuation of the ductus epididymis. In some species, the terminal portion widens to form the ampulla. The ductus deferens terminates at the urethra. Pseudostratified epithelium with microvilli lines the ductus deferens which is also characterized by a thick tunica muscularis of layered smooth muscle.

Accessory Glands

Ampullary glands are absent in the cat and poorly developed in the pig. In other species, the glands form sac-like dilations in the wall of the terminal ductus deferens. The dilations are lined by simple columnar epithelium.

Infoldings of pseudostratified columnar epithelium characterize the **vesicular gland** (seminal vesicle). The glandular lumen contains secretory product but spermatozoa are rarely present. The vesicular gland is not present in the dog or cat.

Secretory units of the **prostate** are lined by pseudostratified epithelium and are surrounded by smooth muscle. Prostatic parenchyma is either compact (carnivores and horse) or disseminate (ox and pig). The prostate surrounds the urethra.

The **bulbourethral gland** (Cowper's gland) has a mucous epithelium. The gland is not present in the dog.

Male Penis and Urethra

The penis consists of the root, body, glans and prepuce. The **glans penis** is covered with stratified squamous epithelium which reflects on the inner surface of the **prepuce** where numerous sweat and sebaceous glands are present. A **tunica albuginea** of dense connective tissue lies beneath the epithelium, and cavernous spaces between the connective tissue trabeculae form erectile tissue. Bone (os penis) is present in some species. The external layer of the prepuce is typical skin.

The male urethra has prostatic, membranous and spongiose regions. The **prostatic portion** extends from the bladder to the prostate and is surrounded by prostatic glandular tissue. The **membranous portion** extends from the prostate to the bulb of the penis. Erectile tissue (corpus spongiosum) envelopes the **spongiose portion** from the bulb to the external opening. The urethra is lined by transitional epithelium. Submucosal glands, erectile tissue and smooth muscle are present in the wall of the urethra.

Scrotum

The external surface of the **scrotum** is a thick skin with hair, sebaceous and sweat glands. The underlying dermis rests on a hypodermis (tunica dartos) with smooth muscle which contracts upon thermal or mechanical stimulation. The **vaginal process,** an evaginated pouch of peritoneum within the scrotum, forms the parietal and visceral vaginal tunics comprised of mesothelium and connective tissue.

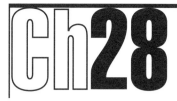

Female Reproductive System

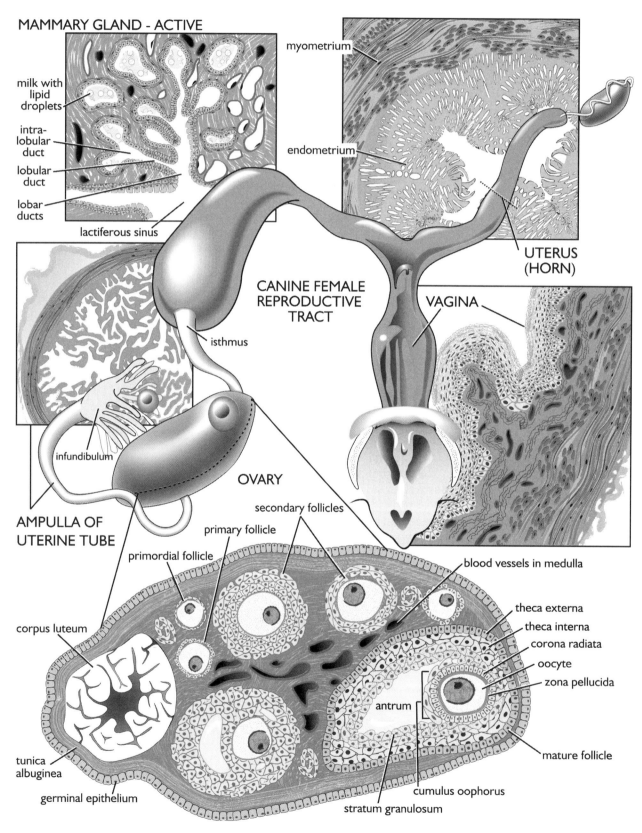

MAMMARY GLAND - ACTIVE

milk with lipid droplets

intra-lobular duct

lobular duct

lobar ducts

lactiferous sinus

myometrium

endometrium

UTERUS (HORN)

CANINE FEMALE REPRODUCTIVE TRACT

isthmus

VAGINA

infundibulum

AMPULLA OF UTERINE TUBE

OVARY

secondary follicles

primary follicle

primordial follicle

corpus luteum

blood vessels in medulla

theca externa

theca interna

corona radiata

oocyte

zona pellucida

antrum

tunica albuginea

germinal epithelium

stratum granulosum

cumulus oophorus

mature follicle

Overview

- The ovary has a cortex containing follicles and a medulla.
- Primordial, primary and secondary follicles have thickening follicular epithelium which develops a central cavity in the mature follicle.
- Atretic follicles regress prior to ovulation while a corpus luteum forms from follicular remnants after ovulation.
- The uterine tube is lined by epithelium with ciliated cells which assist in oocyte transport.
- Endometrium, myometrium and perimetrium are the histologic layers of the uterus.
- The vagina has stratified squamous epithelium which varies with the estrous cycle.

The female reproductive system produces oocytes and endocrine reproductive hormones. If fertilization occurs in the uterine tube, the mammalian conceptus develops in the uterus.

Ovary

A simple cuboidal **germinal epithelium** covers the outer **cortex** of the ovary. Although germ cells migrate through this tissue, they do not arise from the so-called germinal epithelium. The **tunica albuginea,** comprised of dense connective tissue, lies beneath the germinal epithelium. Deeper regions of the cortex contain follicles in various stages of development surrounded by loose connective tissue. **Interstitial endocrine cells** which produce estrogen are present in the stroma of some species. The inner **medulla** of the ovary is loose connective tissue with an extensive vascular supply.

Stage of Follicular Development

The oocyte of a **primordial follicle** is surrounded by a simple squamous epithelium of follicular cells. The follicular cells produce estrogen and are known as **granulosa cells.** At this stage in development, the oocyte is suspended in prophase of the first meiotic division until after ovulation.

Primary follicle stage is reached when follicular epithelium becomes simple cuboidal. Continued development results in a **secondary follicle** with stratified epithelium and a glycoprotein coat around the oocyte called the **zona pellucida.** At this time, connective tissue around the follicle differentiates into the **theca interna** which produces androgens, and the supportive **theca externa.**

Late in follicular development, a central cavity, the **antrum,** forms between the granulosa cells of the **mature follicle. Liquor folliculi,** an oocyte transport fluid, fills the antrum which is lined by the **stratum granulosum.** The oocyte, surrounded by the single cell layer of the **corona radiata,** rests in an accumulation of granulosa cells called the **cumulus oophorus.**

Many follicles regress before ovulation occurs. Pre-ovulatory **atretic follicles** are formed when either the granulosa and thecal cells fill the follicular space or the fluid-filled antrum remains as a cyst.

Following ovulation, the ruptured follicle is filled with blood and is termed a **corpus hermorrhagicum.** Over time, the blood clot is replaced by cells from the stratum granulosum and theca interna to form the **corpus luteum** which produces progesterone and relaxin. The **corpus albicans** is scar tissue which remains after the corpus luteum regresses.

Uterine Tube

The uterine tube extends from the ovary to the uterus. Simple columnar or pseudostratified epithelium with a mixed population of ciliated and microvillous cells lines the tube. A propria-submucosa of connective tissue, a tunica muscularis of smooth muscle, and a tunica serosa are present.

Near the ovary, the **infundibulum** region of the tube has projections which sweep over the surface of the ovary to capture the ovulated oocyte. The **ampulla** has a highly folded tunica mucosa-submucosa, while the **isthmus** region near the uterus has a prominent tunica muscularis which aides the transport of spermatozoa.

Uterus

The uterus is the site of implantation for the fertilized zygote. The inner layer, the **endometrium,** is lined by simple columnar epithelium. Uterine glands are present in the propria-submucosa. Inner circular and outer longitudinal layers of smooth muscle form the **myometrium** which increases considerably during pregnancy. The outer layer of the uterus, the **perimetrium,** is comprised of loose connective tissue covered by mesothelium.

Simple columnar epithelium with mucin-producing cells lines the **cervix.** Smooth muscle and elastic fibers help reestablish cervical structure after parturition.

Vagina

The vagina, a muscular tube extending from the cervix to the vestibule, is lined by stratified squamous epithelium. Epithelial cell characteristics change with the estrous cycle. The tunica muscularis of smooth muscle is surrounded by a typical tunica serosa or adventitia.

Mammary Gland

The mammary gland is a compound tubuloalveolar gland. Simple cuboidal epithelium lines the **secretory alveoli** which are surrounded by myoepithelial cells. Milk flows from the alveolus through the **intralobular duct** to **lobular** and then **lactiferous** (lobar) **ducts.** The milk then collects in the **lactiferous sinus** (gland sinus), exits into the **teat sinus** and then the **papillary duct** (teat canal). Epithelium lining the duct passages transitions from simple cuboidal to stratified squamous at the level of the papillary duct

Corpora amylacea, laminated bodies of degenerated cells or proteins, may be present in the alveoli in advanced milk production.

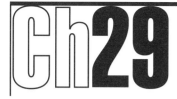

Placentation

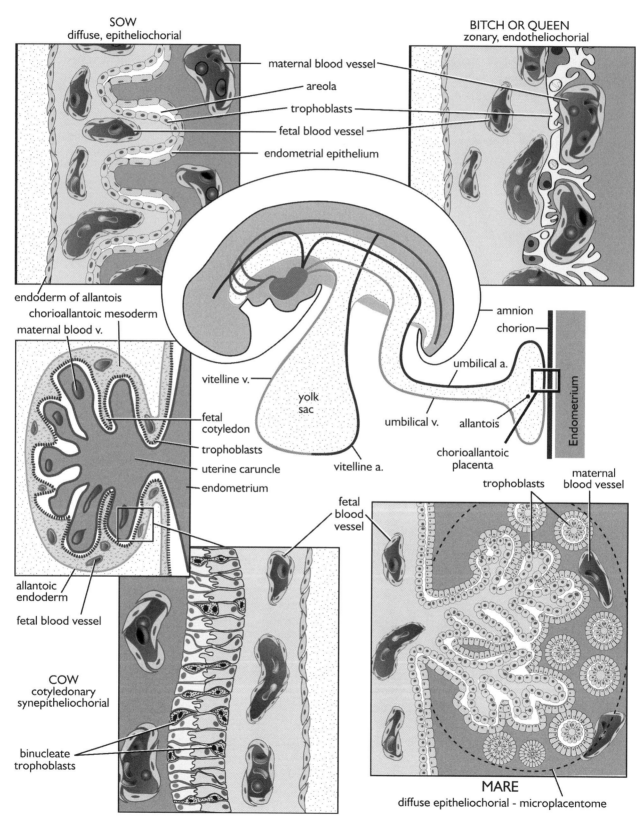

SOW
diffuse, epitheliochorial

maternal blood vessel
areola
trophoblasts
fetal blood vessel
endometrial epithelium

BITCH OR QUEEN
zonary, endotheliochorial

endoderm of allantois
chorioallantoic mesoderm
maternal blood v.

fetal cotyledon
trophoblasts
uterine caruncle
endometrium

allantoic endoderm

fetal blood vessel

vitelline v.

yolk sac

fetal cotyledon

vitelline a.

amnion
chorion

umbilical a.

umbilical v.   allantois

chorioallantoic placenta

Endometrium

fetal blood vessel

trophoblasts   maternal blood vessel

COW
cotyledonary
synepitheliochorial

binucleate trophoblasts

MARE
diffuse epitheliochorial - microplacentome

Overview

- Early choriovitelline placentation is replaced by chorioallantoic placentation in domestic mammals.
- Placental attachment is classified as diffuse, cotyledonary, zonary or discoid.
- A placentome is comprised of a fetal cotyledon and a maternal caruncle.
- The placental barrier includes fetal endothelium, mesenchyme and trophoblasts plus maternal epithelium, connective tissue and endothelium. Components of the barrier vary with the species.
- Types of placentation, based on the number of layers present, include epitheliochorial, syndesmochorial, endotheliochorial and hemochorial.
- Areolae, microplacentomes, endometrial cups and marginal hematomas are species-specific structures associated with placentation.

The mammalian placenta is formed by contact between the fetal extraembryonic membranes and the maternal uterine endometrium.

Choriovitelline and Chorioallantoic Placentation

In choriovitelline placentation, the yolk sac fuses with the chorion and contacts the endometrium to form the placenta during early gestation. This type of placentation is transient and involutes rapidly to be replaced by chorioallantoic placentation in domestic animals. The allantois fuses with the chorion to form the chorioallantoic membrane. The fused extraembryonic membranes contact the endometrium to establish placentation for the remainder of gestation.

Placental Attachment and Shape

In the sow and mare, the fetal chorion forms a highly folded, uniform attachment to the maternal endometrium, described as **diffuse placentation. Cotyledonary placentation** in the ruminant involves isolated tufts of chorion called **cotyledons.** The cotyledons attach to scattered sponge-like uterine caruncles to form placentomes. In carnivores, the chorion forms a villous band around the chorionic sac. The band is the site of uterine attachment in **zonary** placentation. Primates and rodents have a disc of chorion which attaches to the endometrium to create **discoid placentation.**

Layers of the Maternal-Fetal Placental Barrier

The fetal layers of the placental barrier include the **endothelium** of allantoic blood vessels, **mesenchyme** from chorioallantoic mesoderm and **trophoblasts** derived from chorionic ectoderm. Maternal layers are the uterine **endometrial epithelium,** underlying **connective tissue** and **endothelium** of maternal blood vessels.

The number of fetal layers in the placental barrier is constant across domestic species, but the number of maternal layers is variable, depending on the degree of invasion by fetal trophoblasts. In **epitheliochorial** placentation, all three maternal layers persist. Some maternal tissue is lost in **synepitheliochorial placentation.** Trophoblasts fuse as syncytial cells, and some of the binucleate cells erode through the endometrial epithelium to contact maternal connective tissue. In **endotheliochorial** placentation, trophoblasts invade further through the uterine epithelium and connective tissue to contact maternal blood vessels. All three maternal layers are removed, and trophoblasts contact maternal blood in **hemochorial** placentation.

Highly invasive placentation which results in the loss of considerable maternal tissue at parturition is referred to as **deciduate placentation.** Large **deciduate cells** of unknown function are present in the maternal uterine connective tissue. In contrast, little maternal tissue is lost at parturition in **non-deciduate** placentation.

Species Variations in Placentation

The porcine placenta has fluid-filled cups called **areolae** between the trophoblasts and the maternal epithelium. These structures form opposite the openings of endometrial glands and contain glandular secretions.

Focal attachment areas called **microplacentomes** are present in the placenta of the mare. Microscopic villous areas of the chorioallantois attach to the endometrium in a diffuse fashion, and the resulting structures resemble the larger placentome of ruminants. Areolae similar to those in the sow placenta are present between microplacentomes.

At the junction of the chorioallantois and yolk sac in the mare, trophoblasts proliferate and form the **chorionic girdle.** Fetal cells invade the endometrium near the chorionic girdle at 36-38 days of gestation, and form **endometrial cups.** The large cells of the cup produce horse chorionic gonadotropin. Endometrial cups regress after 80 days of gestation.

Hippomanes are free-floating calcified bodies in the allantois which are thought to be cellular debris. The hippomanes are most prominent in horses, but they have also been noted in the pig and ruminant.

White, oval projections on the inner surface of the amnion in horses and ruminants are called **amniotic plaques.** Their function is unknown.

Marginal hematomas are present on the edges of the canine and feline zonary placentae. Maternal endometrium degenerates and hemorrhages as the placenta develops, followed by the formation of a brown or green hematoma.

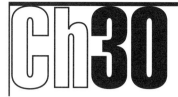

Oral Cavity

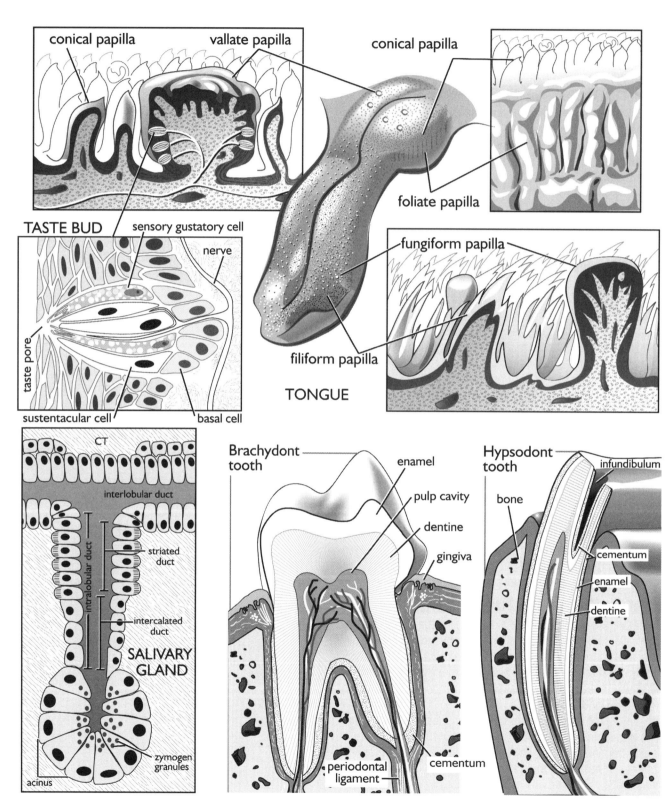

conical papilla   vallate papilla

conical papilla

foliate papilla

TASTE BUD

sensory gustatory cell

nerve

taste pore

sustentacular cell   basal cell

fungiform papilla

filiform papilla

TONGUE

CT

interlobular duct

intralobular duct

striated duct

intercalated duct

SALIVARY GLAND

zymogen granules

acinus

Brachydont tooth

enamel

pulp cavity

dentine

gingiva

cementum

periodontal ligament

Hypsodont tooth

bone

infundibulum

cementum

enamel

dentine

Overview

- The inner lips and cheeks are mucous membranes.
- Stratified squamous epithelium covers the oral surface of the palates while respiratory epithelium lines the nasal surface.
- The dorsal surface of the tongue has lingual papillae.
- Taste buds are present on fungiform, foliate and vallate papillae.
- Enamel and dentine form the crown of branchydont teeth while cementum covers the roots.
- Hyposodont teeth continually grow and their enamel is covered by cementum throughout the length of the tooth.
- Salivary glands are serous, mucous or mixed and are characterized by striated ducts.

The lips, cheeks and palates surround the oral cavity which contains the tongue and teeth. Salivary glands secrete saliva which aides the digestion and passage of food.

Lips and Cheeks

The lips and cheeks are folds of tissue with skin on the external surface and mucous membrane adjacent to the oral cavity. The mucous membrane is stratified squamous epithelium which is keratinized in the ruminant and horse. Underlying connective tissue contains serous or mixed glands and skeletal muscle.

Hard and Soft Palates

The **hard palate** has a keratinized stratified squamous epithelium on the surface with underlying connective tissue that blends with the periosteum of palate bones. The **dental pad,** which functions in place of upper incisors in ruminants, has very thick keratin. Further caudally in the oral cavity, the **soft palate** is present as a fold of mucous membrane with respiratory epithelium on the nasal side and stratified squamous epithelium on the oral side. Aggregated lymphatic tissue is present as the **palatine tonsil.**

Tongue

The dorsal epithelium of the tongue is stratified squamous epithelium with varying degrees of keratinization while ventral epithelium is thin and non-keratinized. The epithelium and underlying connective tissue forms projections on the dorsal surface of the tongue known collectively as **lingual papillae. Filiform papillae** are thorn-shaped and most numerous. **Conical papillae** on the root of the tongue are larger than the filiform papillae and not as heavily keratinized. **Lenticular papillae** are flattened projections found on the ruminant tongue. **Taste buds** are present on the mushroom-shaped **fungiform papillae,** large **vallate papillae,** and in the sides of the grooves of the **foliate folds.** Taste buds are intraepithelial structures which are sensitive for taste. **Sensory gustatory cells** of the taste bud convert chemical molecules into neural impulses which travel along neurons to higher centers in the brain for interpretation as sweet, sour or salty tastes. The **sustentacular cells** of the taste bud are supportive, while the **basal cells** are thought to be precursor cells.

Skeletal muscle and connective tissue forms the central core of the tongue. The skeletal muscle fibers are organized longitudinally, transversely and vertically to give the tongue extensive mobility. A **lyssa** of dense connective tissue in carnivores or bone in the avian is located in the connective tissue on the midline.

Teeth

Enamel, the hardest substance in the body, forms the outer surface of the **crown** of brachydont teeth. **Dentine,** comprised of tubules of collagen fibers and mineral, lies deep to the enamel. The crown narrows and becomes the **neck** region of the tooth just below the gingival surface. The **gingival sulcus** is a space between the neck of the tooth and surrounding gingiva. **Cementum,** also made of collagen and mineral, covers the outer surface of the tooth **root.** A **periodontal ligament** anchors the tooth root to surrounding connective tissue and bone. The central **pulp cavity** of the tooth contains connective tissue, blood vessels and nerves.

During tooth development, enamel is formed by **enameloblasts** (ameloblasts), dentine by **odontoblasts** and cementum by **cementoblasts.** Once the tooth reaches maturity, enameloblasts disappear.

Hypsodont teeth continue to grow throughout life and therefore lack a crown and neck. All equine teeth, the porcine canine tooth and some bovine teeth are hypsodont type. The outer surface of hypsodont teeth is formed by cementum which overlies the enamel. In the center of equine teeth, the cementum invaginates into the enamel and dentine to form the infundibulum in the center of the tooth.

Salivary Glands

The secretory adenomeres of salivary glands are classified as serous, mucous or mixed, based on the epithelial cell types. **Serous** cells contain apical, acidophilic **zymogen granules** which are the stored protein and polysaccharide precursors of saliva. **Mucous** cells have light-staining cytoplasm and a basal nucleus. **Mixed** adenomeres can have either intermixed regions of serous and mucous cells or mucous cells with surrounding **serous demilunes. Myoepithelial cells** surround the secretory units and can contract to assist discharge of the saliva into the duct system.

The intralobular portion of the salivary gland duct system begins with a short **intercalated duct,** lined by simple cuboidal epithelium. The epithelium continues as simple columnar epithelium with extensive basal plasma membrane infoldings in the **striated duct.** Striated ducts are unique to the salivary gland duct system.

The striated ducts empty into **interlobular ducts** followed by **lobular ducts.** Epithelium height increases from simple to stratified columnar in the larger ducts.

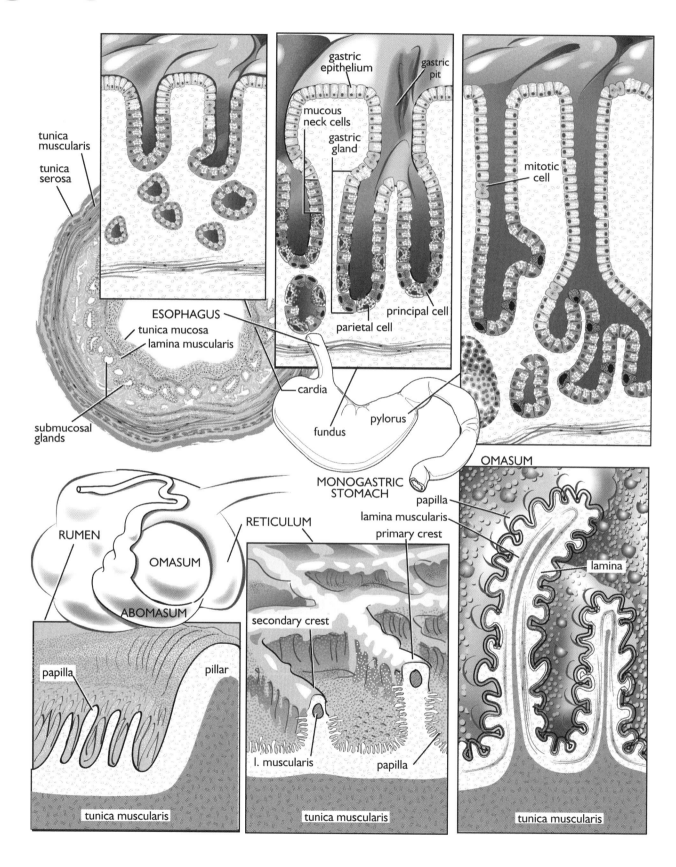

tunica
muscularis

tunica
serosa

ESOPHAGUS
tunica mucosa
lamina muscularis

submucosal
glands

gastric
epithelium

gastric
pit

mucous
neck cells

gastric
gland

parietal cell

principal cell

mitotic
cell

cardia

fundus

pylorus

MONOGASTRIC
STOMACH

OMASUM

papilla

lamina muscularis

primary crest

lamina

RUMEN

OMASUM

RETICULUM

ABOMASUM

secondary crest

papilla

pillar

l. muscularis

papilla

tunica muscularis

tunica muscularis

tunica muscularis

Overview

- The esophagus is lined with stratified squamous epithelium and has smooth, skeletal or mixed smooth muscle in the t. muscularis, depending on the species.
- The stomach is lined by mucus-producing simple columnar epithelium.
- Cardiac glands and pyloric glands have mucous cells.
- Mucous neck cells, principal cells and parietal cells are located in the proper gastric glands.
- The submucosal plexi and myenteric plexi in the t. muscularis supply innervation to the stomach wall.
- The rumen, reticulum and omasum are lined by keratinized stratified squamous epithelium.
- Papillae in the rumen lack a lamina muscularis, small patches of l. muscularis are present in the tips of the crests of the reticulum, and three layers of muscle are present in the laminae of the omasum.

The esophagus transports food from the oral cavity to the stomach. Carnivores, pigs and horses have a monogastric stomach while ruminants have a compound stomach which includes the rumen, reticulum, omasum and abomasum.

Esophagus

The **tunica mucosa** of the esophagus has stratified squamous epithelium adjacent to the lumen. Keratinization of the epithelium increases in relation to increased abrasion from roughage in the diet. Lymphoid tissue often occurs in the lamina propria. The lamina muscularis is comprised of smooth muscle which is inconsistently present. Branched tubuloalveolar seromucous glands are located in the connective tissue of the **tunica submucosa.** The **tunica muscularis** layer may be striated, smooth or mixed muscle types depending on the species. Voluntary striated muscle is present throughout the length of the ruminant and canine esophagus. The porcine esophagus has striated muscle in the cranial portion, mixed muscle types in the thoracic region, and smooth muscle near the stomach. Striated muscle is present in the cranial portion of the feline and equine esophagi, while smooth muscle predominates in the caudal portion. A typical **tunica adventitia** or **tunica serosa** is present as the outer layer.

Monogastric Stomach

The tunica mucosa of the monogastric stomach projects into the lumen as **gastric folds.** Small depressions of the epithelial surface extend into the underlying tissue and are known as **gastric pits.** These pits connect with the lumen of deeper gastric glands.

Mucus-producing simple columnar epithelium forms the lining layer of the stomach. No goblet cells are present in this epithelium. **Cardiac glands** in the lamina propria near the esophagus have short gastric pits and produce mucus. **Proper gastric glands** in the fundus of the stomach have **mucous neck cells** which produce different mucus from surface cells, basophilic **principal cells** (chief cells) which produce pepsinogen, and acidophilic **parietal cells** which secrete hydrochloric acid. **Pyloric glands** are similar in structure to cardiac glands but have deeper gastric pits. A layer of dense connective tissue lies beneath the gastric glands in carnivores and is known as the **stratum compactum.**

The tunica submucosa of the stomach is areolar connective tissue while the tunica muscularis is comprised of inner oblique, middle circular and outer longitudinal layers of smooth muscle. Sympathetic and parasympathetic neuron cell bodies form the **submucosal plexus** (Meissner's plexus), while the **myenteric plexus** (Auerbach's plexus) is located between the middle and outer layers of smooth muscle. These same plexi can also be found in other regions of the tubular digestive tract. A typical tunica serosa is present as the outermost layer of the stomach wall.

The horse has a large non-glandular region between the esophagus and the glandular stomach. This region is demarcated from the glandular stomach by the **margo plicatus** junction, and it is lined by heavily keratinized stratified squamous epithelium. A smaller non-glandular region is present in the pig.

Rumen

The rumen is lined by keratinized stratified squamous epithelium which continues into the reticulum and omasum. Deep cells of the ruminal epithelium play an important role in the metabolism of volatile fatty acids. Glands are absent in the lamina propria.

Pillars of the rumen are large folds of the tunica mucosa which contain smooth muscle from the tunica muscularis. The surface of the pillars is smooth. Conical projections of the mucosa, known as **papillae,** cover the rest of the inner surface of the rumen. The core of a ruminal papilla contains connective tissue but lacks a lamina muscularis.

The tunica muscularis is comprised of layers of smooth muscle which continue in the reticulum, omasum and abomasum. A typical tunica serosa is the outermost layer.

Reticulum

The mucosal folds of the reticulum, or **reticular crests,** form honeycomb-like chambers. **Reticular papillae** are found on the crests and the floor of the chambers. Within the crests, the lamina muscularis is organized as isolated patches of smooth muscle in the tips of the folds.

Omasum

The tunica mucosa of the omasum forms long **omasal laminae** which extend into the lumen. The lamina muscularis and tunica muscularis extend into the core of the laminae to form three layers of smooth muscle. Papillae are present on the surface of the laminae and between laminae.

Abomasum

The lining of the abomasum transitions abruptly to simple columnar epithelium from keratinized stratified squamous found in the non-glandular portions of the compound stomach. Cardiac, fundic and pyloric regions are similar in structure to the analogous regions in the monogastric stomach.

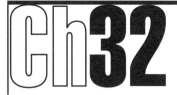

Intestines

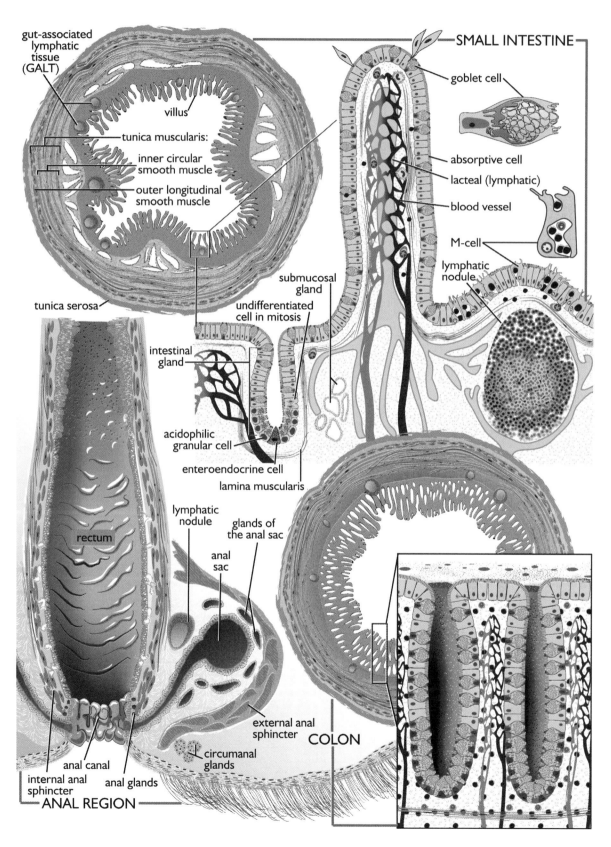

gut-associated lymphatic tissue (GALT)

villus

tunica muscularis:

inner circular smooth muscle

outer longitudinal smooth muscle

tunica serosa

submucosal gland

undifferentiated cell in mitosis

intestinal gland

acidophilic granular cell

enteroendocrine cell

lamina muscularis

SMALL INTESTINE

goblet cell

absorptive cell

lacteal (lymphatic)

blood vessel

M-cell

lymphatic nodule

rectum

lymphatic nodule

glands of the anal sac

anal sac

external anal sphincter

COLON

anal canal

internal anal sphincter

anal glands

circumanal glands

Overview

- The small intestine has villi which are covered by simple columnar epithelium with goblet cells.
- Submucosal glands are present in the initial portion of the small intestine.
- The tunica muscularis of the intestine is organized into inner circular and outer longitudinal layers of smooth muscle.
- Villi are absent in the large intestine and the number of goblet cells in the lining epithelium increases.
- The taeniae, bands of smooth muscle, are present in the tunica muscularis of the cecum and colon.
- The rectum has a venous plexus in the lamina propria.
- Anal glands are modified sweat glands which are separate from the apocrine glands of the anal sac. Nearby circum anal glands are masses of polygonal cells derived from sebaceous glands.

The small intestine includes the duodenum, ileum and jejunum while the cecum, colon and rectum are part of the large intestine. Ingesta passes through the intestine where nutrients and fluids are absorbed, and waste products subsequently pass out of the body.

Small Intestine

Although the regions of the small intestine are defined in gross anatomy of domestic species, histologic differences between the duodenum, ileum and jejunum are not as clear. Therefore these regions of the intestinal tract will be collectively considered as the small intestine.

The mucosa of the small intestine forms **villi** which project into the lumen and greatly increase the overall absorptive surface area of the organ. The surface epithelium of the villi is simple columnar epithelium with numerous goblet cells. **Intestinal absorptive cells** have extensive microvilli on the apical surface. **Goblet cells** are scattered between the absorptive cells and produce mucus. **Intestinal glands** extend from the base of the villi into the underlying lamina propria. Undifferentiated epithelial cells located in the glands divide and migrate up to renew the glandular and surface epithelium every 24-48 hours. **Acidophilic granular cells** (Paneth cells) are present in the epithelium at the base of the glands in ruminants and horses. These cells produce peptidase and lysozyme and may be phagocytic. Enteroendocrine cells are also present in the epithelium of the intestinal glands.

The lamina propria of each villus contains a blind-ended lymphatic capillary, the lacteal. Numerous antibody-producing plasma cells and other cell types are present in the connective tissue surrounding the lacteal.

A lamina muscularis of smooth muscle is located below the lamina propria.

The tunica submucosa is comprised of areolar connective tissue. **Submucosal glands** (Brunner's glands) are mucous in the dog and ruminant, serous in the pig and horse, and mixed seromucous in the cat. Aggregated lymphatic nodules (GALT) are also present in the submucosa along the length of the intestine. The nodules are particularly numerous in the ileal region. Specialized **M cells** which present antigens to the lymphoid tissue are present in the epithelium which overlies the nodules.

The tunica muscularis is characterized by two layers of smooth muscle. The inner layer of circular muscle fibers is surrounded by an outer layer of longitudinal fibers. Orientation of the muscle fibers facilitates peristalsis. Myenteric plexi are often present between muscle layers. A typical tunica serosa lies outside the tunica muscularis as the outermost layer of the organ.

Cecum

The cecum is small in carnivores, but well-developed in herbivores which have a simple stomach. The structure of the cecum is similar to the small intestine except that villi are lacking. Prominent lymphatic nodules are often present in the submucosa. The outer layer of the tunica muscularis has longitudinal bands of smooth muscle, the **taeniae ceci,** which vary in number.

Colon

The colon also lacks mucosal villi. The number of goblet cells in the intestinal epithelium increases significantly to produce more mucus for lubrication as water is absorbed from the intestinal contents in preparation for defecation. **Taeniae coli,** longitudinal bands of smooth muscle, are present in the tunica muscularis of pigs and horses.

Rectum

The structure of the rectum is similar to that of the colon. Goblet cells increase in number and a venous plexus is present in the lamina propria near the anal canal. As the rectum courses retroperitoneally, the tunica serosa changes to a tunica adventitia.

Anal Canal and Associated Glands

The anal canal extends from the rectum to the external anal opening. Lining epithelium transitions from simple columnar epithelium with goblet cells in the colon to stratified squamous epithelium. The **internal anal sphincter** is comprised of smooth muscle from the tunica muscularis layer while the **external anal sphincter** is skeletal muscle.

Anal glands are modified tubuloalveolar sweat glands in the submucosa of the anal region. These glands open into the anal canal along its length. In carnivores, **anal sacs** are paired diverticula of the anus which are lined with stratified squamous epithelium. Associated apocrine **glands of the anal sac** empty into the duct near a sac. Glandular secretions are stored in the sac and released into the anal canal. **Circumanal glands** are small masses of polygonal cells derived from sebaceous glands of the anal region. The ducts of these glands are not patent. Circumanal glands are of clinical concern as they are frequently neoplastic in the dog.

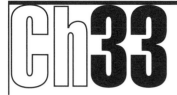

Liver and Gallbladder

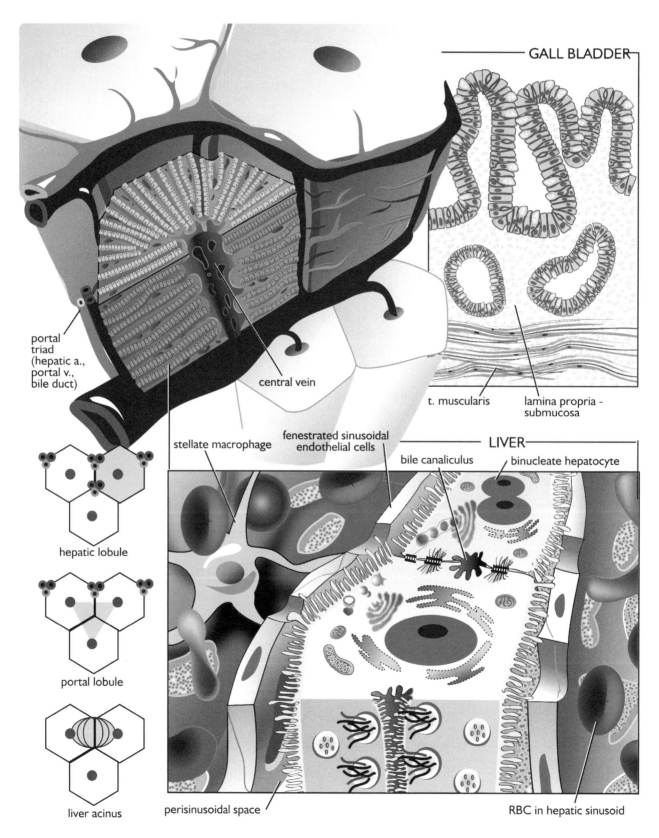

GALL BLADDER

portal triad (hepatic a., portal v., bile duct)

central vein

t. muscularis

lamina propria - submucosa

hepatic lobule

portal lobule

liver acinus

stellate macrophage

fenestrated sinusoidal endothelial cells

LIVER

bile canaliculus

binucleate hepatocyte

perisinusoidal space

RBC in hepatic sinusoid

Overview

- Hepatocytes are large, polyhedral cells with a central nucleus.
- The bile canaliculus is formed by lateral cell membranes of two adjacent hepatocytes.
- Sinusoids are lined by fenestrated endothelial cells and spanned by stellate macrophages.
- In the liver, bile flows through the bile canaliculus, bile ductule, interlobular and intrahepatic bile ducts.
- The portal triad is comprised of a bile duct and branches of the hepatic artery and the portal vein.
- Three conceptual patterns of hepatic tissue arrangement include the hepatic lobule, portal lobule and liver acinus.
- The gallbladder is lined by simple columnar epithelium.

The liver biotransforms toxic substances, secretes bile, synthesizes plasma proteins and clotting factors along with lipids and ketones, stores vitamins and glycogen and is a site of hemopoiesis in the fetus. Bile is stored in the gallbladder, a sac located between the lobes of the liver. The gallbladder is absent in horses.

Capsule and Connective Tissue of the Liver

The **lobes** of the liver are surrounded by a dense irregular connective tissue capsule. The capsule extends into the hepatic parenchyma as areolar connective tissue which separates individual liver **lobules.** Of the domestic species, the porcine liver has the greatest amount of interlobular connective tissue. In other species, the structural lobules are not as clearly defined.

Parenchyma of the Liver

The principal cell of the liver, the **hepatocyte,** is a large, polyhedral cell with a prominent centrally-located nucleus. The cytoplasm contains granular and agranular endoplasmic reticulum, mitochondria and a Golgi apparatus. Microvilli extend from the free surface of the cell, while the lateral surfaces are joined to adjacent hepatocytes by desmosomes and gap junctions. An indentation in the lateral cell membrane of two adjacent hepatocytes forms a tube-like structure between the cells called the **bile canaliculus.** Microvilli extend into the lumen of the canaliculus.

Hepatocytes are arranged as plates of cells which radiate from a central vein within each hepatic lobule. Vascular sinusoids ramify between the plates and are lined by **sinusoidal endothelial cells.** The endothelial cells are fenestrated and have numerous pores. Phagocytic **stellate macrophage cells** (Kupffer cells) extend across the lumen of the sinusoids. The endothelial cells are separated from the surface of the underlying hepatocytes by a narrow **perisinusoidal space** (space of Disse). Tissue fluid can exit the sinusoid across the endothelium to bathe the hepatocytes, but blood cells are retained in circulation.

Biliary and Blood Flow in the Liver

Bile flows from the hepatocyte where it is produced into the **bile canaliculus,** and then into the **bile ductule** which is lined by low, simple cuboidal epithelium. Bile then enters the **interlobular ducts** followed by **intrahepatic** and **extrahepatic bile ducts.** The lining epithelium increases in height from simple cuboidal in the interlobular ducts to simple columnar epithelium in the later ducts.

In the interlobular connective tissue, the **bile duct,** and branches of the **hepatic artery** and **portal vein** are collectively referred to as the **portal triad.** Blood travels in one direction in the portal triad vessels, while bile travels in the opposite direction in the biliary system.

Blood flows from both the hepatic artery and the portal vein into the hepatic sinusoids. After percolating through the sinusoids, the blood exits the lobule through the **central vein** into the sublobular vein and finally into the hepatic vein.

Hepatic Units

Three different conceptual patterns of hepatic tissue arrangement are proposed, based on morphology, exocrine function or vascular supply. Tissue of the **hepatic lobule** is arranged around the central vein with portal triads forming the peripheral boundaries of the lobule. The interlobular bile duct in the portal triad is the center of the **portal lobule,** with central veins forming the corners of the portal lobule. The **liver acinus** is organized around interlobular vessels and represents zones of adjacent lobules which are supplied by the same blood vessel. Zone one receives the freshest blood with the highest concentration of nutrients and oxygen, however cells in this zone are also the first to be exposed to any entering toxins. Zone three is furthest from the incoming blood.

Gallbladder

When the gallbladder is contracted, the inner mucosa is highly folded. The lamina epithelialis of the mucosa is simple columnar epithelium. Goblet cells are present in the epithelium of the ruminant gallbladder. The gallbladder epithelium invaginates as sinuses into the connective tissue of the underlying propria-submucosa, and these invaginations are sometimes mistaken for glands. Randomly-arranged smooth muscle forms the tunica muscularis and a typical tunica serosa covers the outer surface of the gallbladder.

Bile exits the liver in the **hepatic bile duct,** and then flows into the **cystic bile duct** to the gallbladder where it is stored and concentrated. Bile leaving the gallbladder flows out through the cystic bile duct in the opposite direction. The cystic bile duct joins the hepatic bile duct to form the **common bile duct** which empties into the duodenum.

The wall of the **bile ducts** is similar in structure to the wall of the gallbladder, but the smooth muscle in the tunica muscularis of the ducts is arranged in inner circular and outer longitudinal layers. Near the entrance to the duodenum, the smooth muscle of the common bile duct thickens to form the **bile duct sphincter** which controls bile flow into the duodenum.

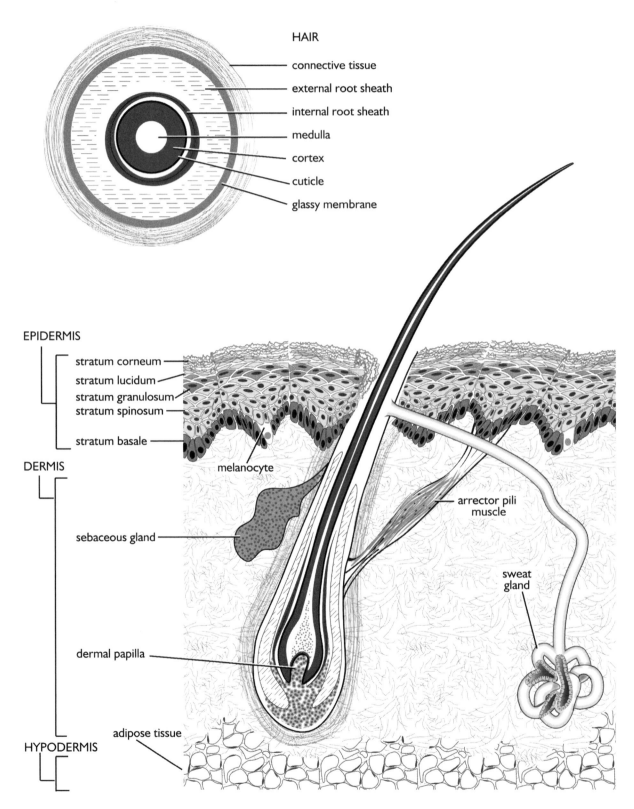

HAIR
- connective tissue
- external root sheath
- internal root sheath
- medulla
- cortex
- cuticle
- glassy membrane

EPIDERMIS
- stratum corneum
- stratum lucidum
- stratum granulosum
- stratum spinosum
- stratum basale

melanocyte

DERMIS

sebaceous gland

arrector pili muscle

sweat gland

dermal papilla

HYPODERMIS

adipose tissue

Overview

- The skin is comprised of the epidermis, dermis and hypodermis.
- Layers of the epidermis include the stratum corneum, stratum lucidum, stratum spinosum, and stratum basale.
- Keratinocytes are the principal cell of the epidermis.
- Sebaceous glands are associated with hair follicles.
- Apocrine sweat glands are prominent in horse skin.
- The internal and external root sheaths of the hair follicle are surrounded by a glassy membrane.
- Anagen, catagen and telogen are stages of the hair cycle.
- The horn, chestnut and ergot are comprised of tubular and intertubular horn.

Skin covers the outer surface of the body and protects underlying structures. In addition, skin serves as a protective barrier, a sensory and thermoregulatory organ, and a participant in the immune response. In many species, skin is modified into structures which provide species recognition and adornment.

Skin

The skin is comprised of the epidermis, dermis and hypodermis. The **epidermis** is stratified squamous epithelium of varying thickness with varying amounts of keratinization.

The upper keratinized layer of the epidermis, the **stratum corneum,** is comprised of several layers of anucleate, squamous cells which contain large amounts of fibrous **keratin** and **keratohyalin** granules.

The **stratum lucidum** is formed by several layers of translucent squamous cells which stain palely and are devoid of both nucleus and organelles. Eleidin is present in the cells of this layer. The stratum lucidum is prominent in the footpads, nose and periople of the hoof.

Basophilic keratohyalin granules and lamellar granules are identifying features of the cells of the **stratum granulosum.**

Cells in the **stratum spinosum** have numerous intercellular bridges (desmosomes) which result in a spiny appearance of the fixed cells. Tonofilaments are formed in this layer.

The **stratum basale** is the deepest layer of the epidermis. Cells in this layer either divide to form the layers above or anchor the epidermis to the underlying dermis.

Keratinocytes are the principal epithelial cell of the epidermis. In the deeper epithelial layers, the keratinocyte may be pigmented. **Melanocytes** are clear cells which produce melanin and transfer it in membrane-bounded **melanosomes** to the keratinocytes. **Intraepidermal macrophages** (Langerhan's cells) are located in the granular cell layer and present antigen to lymphocytes as a component of the cutaneous immune response. **Tactile epithelial cells** (Merkel cells) synapse with sensory axons in the basal layers of the epidermis and are thought to be mechanoreceptors.

The **dermis** varies from loose to dense connective tissue with a rich population of fibroblasts, fibrocytes, macrophages and mast cells. The **papillary zone** interdigitates with the basal region of the epidermis to anchor the skin. Dense connective tissue of the **reticular zone** of the dermis is arranged in bundles along lines of tension.

The **hypodermis** is areolar connective tissue with a variable amount of adipose tissue infiltration. This layer attaches the skin to underlying structures.

Glands Associated with Skin

Sebaceous glands are associated with hair follicles in skin. Apocrine sweat glands are the principal sweat gland of animal skin, and are very active in the horse. Merocine sweat glands are located in the footpad of carnivores, the frog of the horse, and the nasolabial region of ruminants and swine. The secretions of the sebaceous and sweat glands help lubricate, moisturize and cool the integument.

Hair

Hair is formed in a **hair follicle** which is an invagination of the epidermis into the underlying dermis. A **glassy membrane** separates the follicular epithelium from the surrounding connective tissue. The **external root sheath** and **internal root sheath** form the balance of the hair follicle wall. A hair develops from cells in the periphery of the **dermal papilla,** located in the floor of the hair follicle.

The **hair bulb** is an enlarged region of the hair located over the dermal papilla. A **cuticle** forms the outer surface of the hair and has a unique pattern ranging from smooth to scaly. The **cortex,** located beneath the cuticle, is often pigmented and imparts color to the hair. An air-filled space in the center of the hair called the **medulla,** is absent from secondary hairs.

A thin strip of smooth muscle, the **arrector pili muscle,** originates from the epidermis near each follicle and inserts on the follicular wall. The muscle contracts under the influence of sympathetic innervation and erects the hair.

The follicles of large **sensory hairs** (whiskers) are surrounded by vascular sinuses containing blood, dense connective tissue, and free and tactile nerve endings.

The hair cycle begins with **anagen,** a period of growth. Shedding occurs during early anagen. Anagen is followed by **catagen,** at which time the cells in the hair bulb regress and separate from the papillae. During **telogen,** the long resting stage, a secondary hair germ develops in preparation for a repeat of the cycle.

Horn, Chestnut and Ergot

The horns of oxen are bony prominences of the skull covered by hard keratinized epidermis. Tubular and intertubular horn make up the stratum corneum of the horn.

In the horse, the chestnut and ergot are vestiges of carpal and metacarpal pads that are comprised of tubular and intertubular horn.

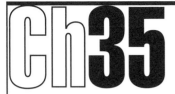

Hoof and Claw

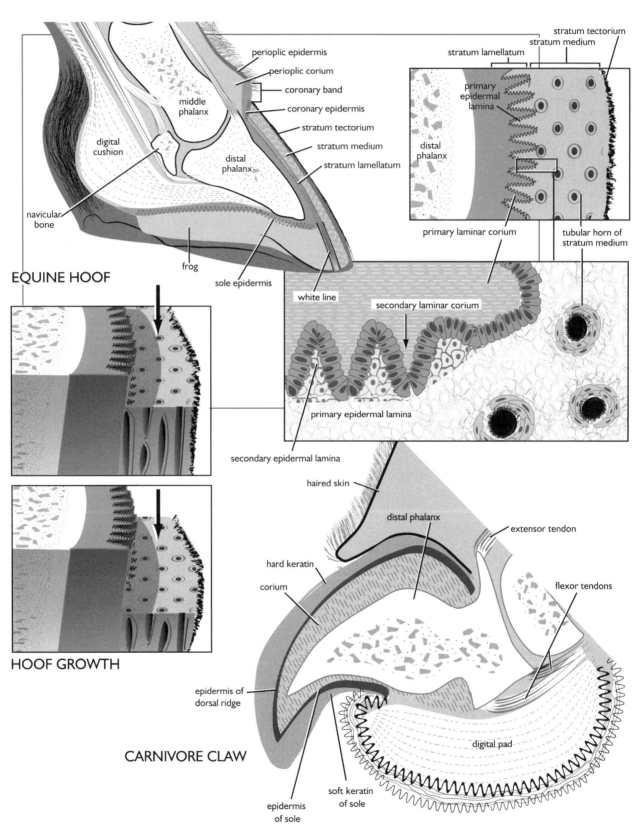

EQUINE HOOF

- perioplic epidermis
- perioplic corium
- coronary band
- coronary epidermis
- stratum tectorium
- stratum medium
- stratum lamellatum

middle phalanx

digital cushion

distal phalanx

navicular bone

frog

sole epidermis

HOOF GROWTH

stratum tectorium
stratum medium
stratum lamellatum

primary epidermal lamina

distal phalanx

primary laminar corium

tubular horn of stratum medium

white line

secondary laminar corium

primary epidermal lamina

secondary epidermal lamina

haired skin

distal phalanx

extensor tendon

hard keratin

flexor tendons

corium

epidermis of dorsal ridge

digital pad

CARNIVORE CLAW

epidermis of sole

soft keratin of sole

Overview

- The epidermis of the periople and the coronary band gives rise to outer layers of the hoof wall.
- A corium of connective tissue underlies the epidermis of the hoof.
- The hoof wall is comprised of the thin stratum tectorium from the perioplic epidermis, a stratum medium of tubular and intertubular horn from the coronary epidermis and a stratum lamellatum of interdigitating laminar epidermis and connective tissue.
- The stratum lamellatum of the equine hoof has primary and secondary laminae while ruminant and porcine hooves have primary laminae only.
- Hard keratin comprises the wall and dorsal ridge of the carnivore claw while soft keratin forms the sole.

The equine, bovine and porcine hooves and the carnivore claw are modified from skin. They each surround the bone of the digit and are important in locomotion.

Equine Hoof

The hoof has an **epidermis** and a connective tissue corium which is continuous with the epidermis and dermis of the haired skin of the leg. A thin layer of stratum basale and stratum spinosum plus a thicker stratum corneum form the epidermis. The stratum granulosum and stratum lucidum found in cutaneous skin are not present.

The **periople,** a roll of tissue below the haired skin but above the hoof wall, is comprised of epidermis and corium. Three layers of the **hoof wall** include the stratum tectorium, stratum medium and stratum lamellatum. **Perioplic epidermis** produces the **stratum tectorium** which grows downward to cover the outer surface of the hoof. The papillated **perioplic corium** lies beneath the epidermis and attaches the hoof to underlying structures.

Located just distal to the periople, the **coronary band** is comprised of the coronary epidermis and coronary corium. The **coronary epidermis** angles away from the outer surface of the hoof toward the deep bone of the distal phalanx. Due to the angle of orientation of the epidermis, the keratin layer extends from the surface of the epidermis toward the ground. The keratinized cells of the epidermis are arranged as **tubular** and **intertubular horn** to form the **stratum medium** of the hoof wall. **Coronary corium** is papillated connective tissue beneath the epidermis.

The **stratum lamellatum** is an interdigitating region of epidermis and connective tissue which runs parallel to the anterior surface of the distal phalanx. The coronary epidermis becomes the **laminar epidermis** as it angles down the hoof wall. The epidermis forms primary and secondary laminae which interdigitate with the underlying connective tissue of the **laminar corium.** The **primary epidermal laminae** are nontubular, hard keratin and are considered insensitive laminae. **Secondary epidermal laminae** protrude off the surface of the primary laminae and include the cellular stratum spinosum and stratum basale layers. The secondary epidermal laminae interdigitate with the secondary laminae of the corium which extend off the primary laminar corium. Sensitive laminae include the secondary epidermal laminae and the primary and secondary laminar corium. In addition

to the laminar corium, a dermal layer of corium is present between the stratum lamellatum and the periosteum of the distal phalanx.

The stratum lamellatum is the **white line** of the hoof which is visible on the ground contact surface between the hoof wall and the sole. Horseshoe nails placed outside the white line will be located in insensitive tissue away from the stratum lamellatum.

The epidermis and corium of the bars, sole and frog are similar in structure to the rest of the foot except that the horn is softer. Fibroelastic connective tissue forms the **digital cushion** located between the sole of the hoof and the bones of the foot. The cushion functions in shock absorption and attachment of the hoof.

The hoof wall grows continually and is trimmed or worn away by abrasion with the ground. Epidermal germ cells at the coronary band add new horn to the wall. Clusters of epidermal cells in the secondary laminae detach from the primary laminae periodically and allow the laminae to slide downward toward the ground. New keratin is produced by the stationary cells of the secondary laminae.

Ruminant and Porcine Hooves

The histologic structure of the ruminant and porcine hooves is similar to that of the equine hoof except that secondary laminae of the stratum lamellatum are absent. Primary epidermal laminae are formed by keratin produced from the smooth, overlying layer of epidermal cells. Connective tissue of the corium interdigitates between the primary epidermal laminae.

Carnivore Claw

The claws of dogs and cats consist of two walls and a central dorsal ridge made of hard keratin plus a soft keratin sole. The hard keratin of the walls and ridge originates from the underlying epidermis which is most active in the coronary and ridge regions. Softer sole keratin is produced by the epidermis of the sole. The corium, located between the epidermis and the distal phalanx, is very vascular connective tissue and bleeds profusely when cut.

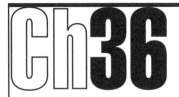
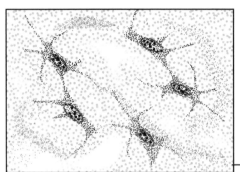

INTRAMEMBRANOUS BONE FORMATION

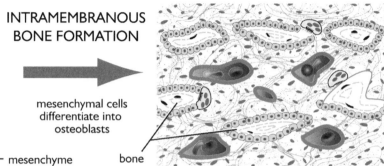

mesenchymal cells differentiate into osteoblasts

— mesenchyme

bone

ENDOCHONDRAL BONE FORMATION

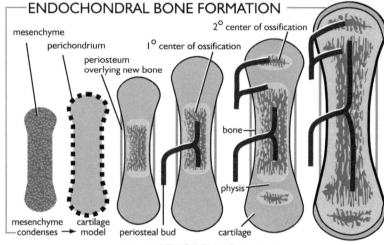

mesenchyme

perichondrium

periosteum overlying new bone

1° center of ossification

2° center of ossification

bone

physis

mesenchyme condenses → cartilage model

periosteal bud

cartilage

GROWTH PLATE

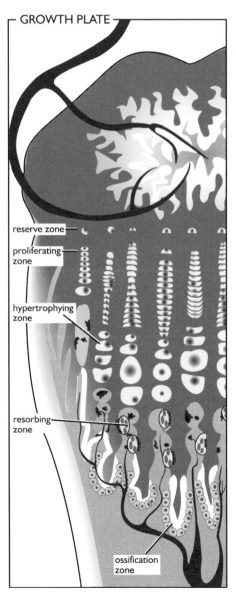

reserve zone

proliferating zone

hypertrophying zone

resorbing zone

ossification zone

REMODELING

spongy bone

compact bone

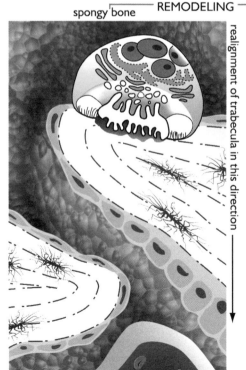

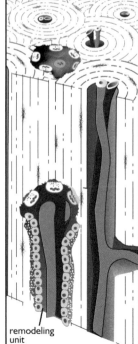

realignment of trabecula in this direction

remodeling unit

Overview

- Cartilage can increase in size by either interstitial or appositional growth; bone can only grow by apposition.
- Intramembranous bone forms in soft tissue; endochondral bone forms within a cartilage model.
- The organization of woven bone is irregular; lamellar bone is deposited in layers.
- Long bone formation begins with mesenchymal condensation followed by a cartilage model, and ends with physeal closure.
- Growth in length of a long bone occurs at the physis.
- Modeling is the change in shape of a long bone while remodeling is the turnover of an adult bone.

Cartilage Development and Growth

Cartilage develops from local mesoderm which is shaped as the adult cartilage or bone it later becomes. The cells aggregate and differentiate into chondroblasts and begin secreting matrix. Connective tissue around the outside of the model is called **perichondrium.** The cartilage model can increase in size by either **interstitial** or **appositional growth.**

Bone Development and Growth

Bone development can be classified by either the precursor tissue or the morphology of the newly formed bone. **Intramembranous bone formation** begins with mesenchymal cells that become osteoblasts and form osteoid within the existing soft tissue. In the case of **endochondral bone formation,** a cartilage precursor model is formed initially. Later, differentiated osteoblasts form osteoid on the surface of a residual calcified cartilage framework. In contrast to cartilage, bone can only grow by apposition of new bone on a surface.

The matrix of **woven bone** has an irregular pattern resembling woven cloth. Woven bone is deposited rapidly and is found in fetal bone, tumors or fracture repair. **Lamellar bone** is deposited in layers and is typical of mature bone.

Stages of Long Bone Formation

Long bone formation begins with the condensation of mesenchyme. Mesenchymal cells become chondroblasts which form matrix. The cartilage model is surrounded by **perichondrium** and resembles the shape of the adult long bone.

As time passes, the central cells of the cartilage model hypertrophy and their surrounding matrix calcifies. On the periphery of the cartilage model, a **periosteal collar** of bone forms. A vascular bud from the periosteum invades the center of the cartilage model, and accompanying osteogenic cells form the bone of the **primary center of ossification.**

The primary center of ossification expands to fill the diaphyseal-metaphyseal region of the long bone. Vascular buds in **cartilage canals** invade the epiphyseal regions of the bone and initiate the formation of one or more **secondary centers of ossification**. The number and time of appearance of the secondary centers varies with the species.

Long Bone Growth and Modeling

Modeling is the change of shape of a growing bone. Modeling occurs concurrently with the increase in size of the immature bone.

The **physis** (cartilaginous growth plate) is responsible for the growth in length of a long bone. Chondrocytes in the physis are arranged in long columns. The **reserve zone** is comprised of resting cells at the top of the columns. This zone anchors the physis to the overlying epiphyseal bone. The **proliferating zone** is the region of active chondrocyte division. Chondrocytes increase in size and the matrix between the columns mineralizes in the **hypertrophying zone.** The terminal chondrocytes in the columns deteriorate as osteoclasts open the lacunae and metaphyseal blood vessels invade in the **resorbing zone.** Osteoblasts accompanying the blood vessels deposit new bone on the remnants of the calcified cartilage in the **ossification zone.** Thus, growth is accomplished by adding new cartilage cells at the top of the physis while bone is formed on cartilage remnants in the metaphysis.

A long bone grows in width by the addition of new bone on the periosteal surface. Concurrently, bone is resorbed on the endosteal surface to widen the marrow cavity and maintain a constant cortical thickness. The shape of the long bone is sculpted by osteoblastic or osteoclastic activity in specific regions, a process called **modeling.** At skeletal maturity, the physis closes as chondrocytes in the proliferating zone cease division, but metaphyseal blood vessels continue their penetration of the cartilage followed by bone formation.

Bone Remodeling

After skeletal maturity, bone continues to turn over in a process called **remodeling.** The trabeculae of spongy bone are remodeled by osteoclastic activity that removes bone on the surface. New bone is then reformed in the same location (replacement) or on the opposite side of the trabecula (realignment) by osteoblasts.

The remodeling unit of compact bone is comprised of a cutting cone of osteoclasts that remove the compact bone. The activity of the cutting cone is followed by a wave of osteoblasts that fill the eroded cavity with bone of a new osteon.

Ch37 Joints

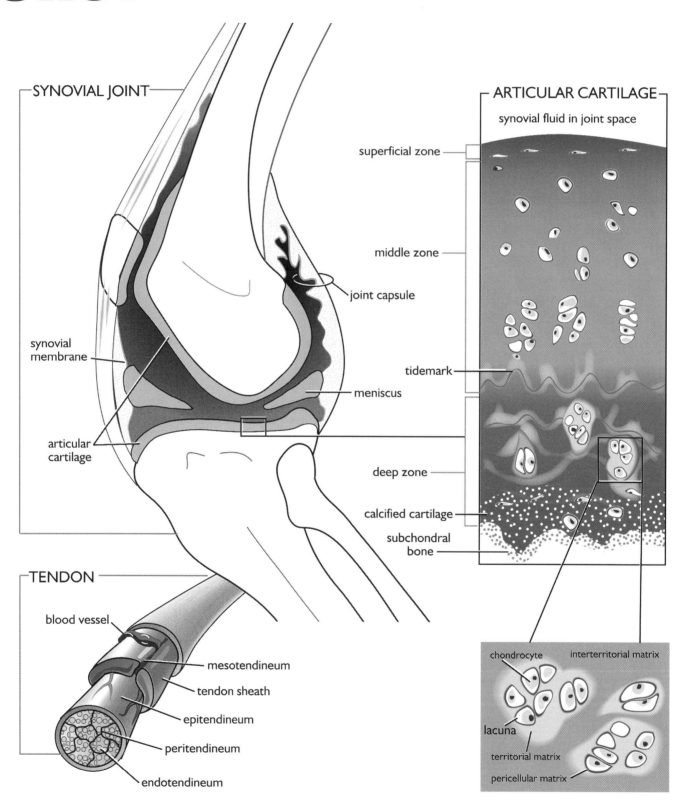

SYNOVIAL JOINT

synovial membrane

articular cartilage

joint capsule

meniscus

ARTICULAR CARTILAGE

synovial fluid in joint space

superficial zone

middle zone

tidemark

deep zone

calcified cartilage

subchondral bone

TENDON

blood vessel

mesotendineum

tendon sheath

epitendineum

peritendineum

endotendineum

chondrocyte

interterritorial matrix

lacuna

territorial matrix

pericellular matrix

Overview

- The bones of fibrous and cartilaginous joints are joined by connective tissue or cartilage.
- A synovial joint has a joint capsule with a lining of synovial membrane which produces synovial fluid found in the joint space.
- Articular cartilage has superficial, middle and deep zones.
- Pericellular, territorial, and interterritorial matrix regions of articular cartilage have different proteoglycans.
- Menisci are fibrocartilage.
- Ligaments and tendons are dense, regular connective tissue.

The musculoskeletal system is comprised of joints, the articulations between two or more bones, and their associated ligaments, tendons and muscles.

Histologic Classification of Joints

A **fibrous joint** which connects two bones together by means of a ligament is a **syndesmoses,** while a joint comprised of connective tissue is known as a **suture.** A cartilaginous joint formed by either hyaline cartilage or fibrocartilage is a **synchondroses** or a **symphysis** respectively. The bones of a **synovial joint** have cartilage on their articulating surfaces. A **joint capsule** surrounds the joint space and contains lubricating **synovial fluid** between the gliding cartilage surfaces. Intraarticular ligaments and menisci may also be present within the synovial joint space.

Joint Capsule and Synovial Membrane

The joint capsule of synovial joints has an outer fibrous layer and an inner synovial membrane layer. The **fibrous layer** is dense irregular connective tissue. **Synovial membrane** lines the inner surface of the joint capsule, and may also form villi or cover over intra-articular ligaments within the joint space.

Spherical or flattened synovial cells lie among connective tissue fibers at the surface of the synovial membrane. **Fibroblast synovial cells** produce the components of synovial fluid, while **macrophage synovial cells** are phagocytic. An **intermediate synovial cell** has characteristics of both fibroblast and macrophage cell types.

Synovial membrane is classified by the connective tissue located beneath the cellular layer. Areolar, fibrous or adipose connective tissue is present at various locations around the joint capsule.

Articular Cartilage

Articular cartilage on the surface of bones is predominately hyaline cartilage however, fibrocartilage is occasionally present in this role.

The **superficial zone** of articular cartilage is adjacent to the joint space and is characterized by flattened chondrocytes. Collagen fibers in the matrix of the superficial zone run parallel with the articular surface. Chondrocytes in the **middle zone** are spherical, and collagen fibers change direction to run perpendicular with the cartilage surface. In the **deep zone,** cells are arranged in clusters or columns. The matrix fibers continue perpendicular with the cartilage surface, and the deeper region of the matrix is calcified. A basophilic line, the **tidemark,** appears between the calcified and non-calcified regions of the deep zone at skeletal maturity. The deep zone anchors the articular cartilage to the underlying subchondral bone.

Staining differences in the matrix of articular cartilage are due largely to differences in density and type of proteoglycans. A dark staining, thin **pericellular matrix** immediately surrounds individual lacunae. **Territorial matrix** is located outside the pericellular matrix, while lighter staining **interterritorial matrix** fills the space between regions of territorial matrix.

As articular cartilage is avascular, nutrients are supplied by diffusion from the synovial fluid which bathes the tissue surface. Calcified cartilage in the deep layer serves as an effective barrier to supply from below by subchondral blood vessels.

Menisci

Menisci are fibrocartilaginous structures which are interposed in the joint space between articular cartilage surfaces. These C-shaped or disc-shaped structures function in load bearing and shock absorption during locomotion.

Ligaments

Ligaments are dense, regular connective tissue bands or cords which join bone to bone. Intracapsular ligaments are located within the joint capsule while extracapsular ligaments are found on the external capsular surface. Fibrocartilage is frequently present at the bony insertion of a ligament. Collagen fibers of the ligament continue into the bone matrix as **perforating fibers** (Sharpey's fibers).

Tendons

Tendons are also dense regular connective tissue, but they connect muscle to bone.

Individual collagen fibers of a tendon are surrounded by connective tissue known as **endotendineum. Peritendineum** is connective tissue which surrounds bundles of collagen fibers. The entire tendon is surrounded by epitendineum.

A **synovial sheath** may be present where a tendon passes through a bony groove. The tendon indents the elongated, sac-like sheath which contains synovial fluid. The inner layer of the sheath is attached to the epitendiuneum. Vessels and nerves enter the tendon between edges of the sheath through an area called the **mesotendineum.**

Synovial Bursa

A **synovial bursa** is a sac-like structure which lies beneath a tendon, ligament or muscle and a bony prominence at a pressure point. Synovial fluid is secreted into the lumen of the bursa by lining cells.

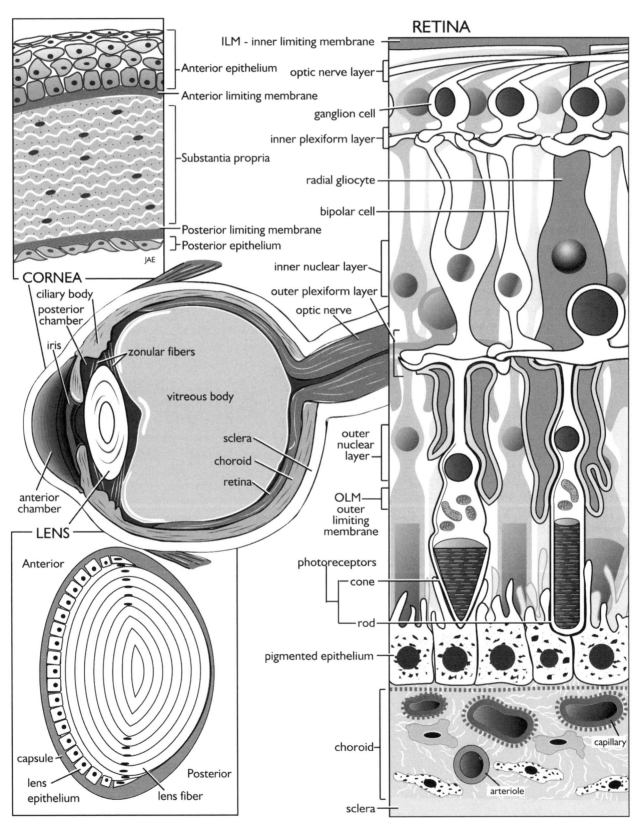

CORNEA

- Anterior epithelium
- Anterior limiting membrane
- Substantia propria
- Posterior limiting membrane
- Posterior epithelium

JAE

LENS

- Anterior
- capsule
- lens epithelium
- lens fiber
- Posterior

ciliary body
posterior chamber
iris
zonular fibers
vitreous body
anterior chamber
sclera
choroid
retina

RETINA

- ILM - inner limiting membrane
- optic nerve layer
- ganglion cell
- inner plexiform layer
- radial gliocyte
- bipolar cell
- inner nuclear layer
- outer plexiform layer
- optic nerve
- outer nuclear layer
- OLM outer limiting membrane
- photoreceptors
  - cone
  - rod
- pigmented epithelium
- choroid
  - capillary
  - arteriole
- sclera

Overview

- The sclera is dense connective tissue.
- Layers of the transparent cornea include the anterior epithelium, anterior limiting membrane, substantia propria, posterior limiting membrane and posterior epithelium.
- The vascular tunic includes the choroid, ciliary body and iris.
- The lens capsule surrounds the epithelium and fibers of the lens.
- The ten histologic layers of the retina include the pigmented epithelium, three neurons, intervening synaptic regions, processes of supporting cells, and axons of the optic nerve.
- The anterior compartment contains aqueous humor while the posterior compartment contains the vitreous body.

The eye gathers and focuses light, and transmits resulting nervous impulses to the brain for interpretation as images.

Fibrous Tunic

The fibrous tunic of the eye includes the sclera and cornea.

The **sclera,** of dense white connective tissue, forms the outer covering of the posterior eye. Bone or cartilage may be present in the sclera of the avian eye.

The **cornea** is the highly transparent outer layer of the anterior eye. The **anterior epithelium** of the cornea is non-keratinized, stratified squamous epithelium which is richly endowed with nerve endings. An **anterior limiting membrane** (Bowman's membrane), composed of a basement membrane and collagen network, is present in primates. The **substantia propria** of the cornea is collagen fibers, which are highly ordered for transparency. A **posterior limiting membrane** (Descemet's membrane) separates the substantia propria from the simple squamous or cuboidal **posterior epithelium** (corneal endothelium).

Vascular Tunic

The vascular tunic lies deep to the sclera and is comprised of the choroid, ciliary body, and iris.

The outer layer of the **choroid** is the **suprachoroid** which is connective tissue. Deep to the suprachoroid is a **vascular layer.** In most domestic species except for the pig, a light reflective layer, the **tapetum lucidum**, is present between the vascular layer and the **choriocapillary layer.** The **basal complex** (Bruch's membrane) separates the capillaries in the choriocapillary layer from the retina.

The **ciliary body** has **ciliary processes** which are covered with two layers of cuboidal epithelium. The deep layer of epithelial cells is pigmented. The ciliary processes produce **aqueous humor. Zonular fibers** extend from the processes and attach to the lens. The smooth **ciliary muscle** at the base of the processes contracts to change the shape of the lens.

The **iris** controls the amount of light entering the eye through the pupil. The anterior surface, or **stratum avascularorum,** is connective tissue rather than epithelium. Pigment in the **stroma** beneath determines the color of the eye. The stroma also contains **pupillary dilator** and **sphincter muscles.** A **posterior surface epithelium** is heavily pigmented.

Lens

The outer surface of the lens is a **capsule** which is the basement membrane of the **lens epithelium.** The epithelium is simple cuboidal and is confined to the anterior surface of the lens underneath the capsule. The epithelial cells elongate to form spindle-shaped **lens fibers** at the equator of the lens. The fibers lose their nuclei and sink toward the center of the lens throughout life. Junction of the fibers forms a Y-shaped **suture** on the anterior lens and an inverted Y suture on the posterior lens surface.

Retina

The retina is comprised of three neurons with intervening synaptic regions. The outer layer is a **pigmented epithelium** of cuboidal cells which protect the photoreceptors above. **Rods and cones** contain rhodopsin and iodopsin, the visual pigment of the eye. These cells shed disks which are phagocytized by the pigmented epithelium. Nuclei of **rods and cones, bipolar cells,** and **ganglion cells** form the nucleated layers of the retina. Processes of radial gliocytes (Müeller cells) form the supporting outer and inner limiting membranes. The outer plexiform layer is the synaptic region between the photoreceptor and bipolar cells, while the inner plexiform layer represents the synapses between the bipolar and ganglion cells. Ganglion cell axons form the optic nerve fiber layer which converges at the optic disk to form the optic nerve which exits to the brain.

Compartments of the Eye

The anterior compartment of the eye contains the anterior chamber which extends from the cornea to the iris, and the posterior chamber which extends from the iris to the lens. Aqueous humor, a fluid produced by the ciliary processes, flows through the iris and drains at the iridial angle between the cornea and iris. The posterior compartment is located between the lens and the retina and contains the vitreous body, a gelatinous structure of hyaluron, collagen and water.

Eyelids, Nictitating Membrane and Lacrimal Gland

The eyelid is a fold of skin with large sebaceous tarsal glands along the margin. Hair is present on the outer surface of the eyelid. A conjunctival fold, the nicitating membrane, contains hyaline or elastic cartilage and lymphatic nodules. The lacrimal gland is mucous in the pig, seromucous in the dog and serous in other domestic species.

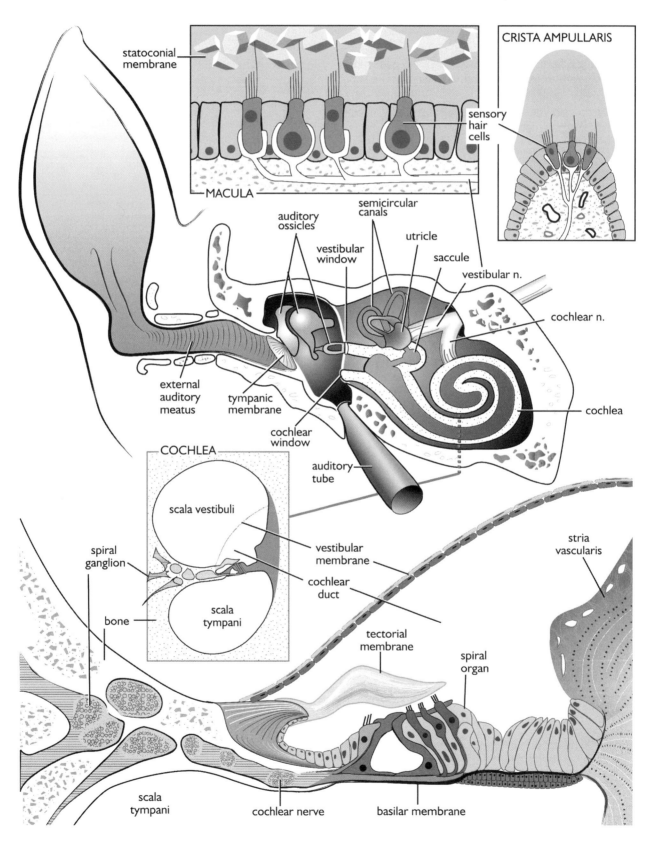

Overview

- The pinna is skin with a cartilaginous core.
- Ceruminous glands are modified sweat glands.
- The tympanic membrane is two layers of epithelium separated by connective tissue.
- Respiratory epithelium lines the auditory tube.
- The vestibular apparatus includes the semicircular canals, ampula, utricle and saccule.
- The crista ampullaris and maculae send neural impulses to the brain via the vestibular nerve.
- The auditory apparatus includes the scala vestibuli, scala tympani and cochlear duct.
- Sensory cells in the spiral organ transmit neural impulses to the auditory nerve for hearing.
- Endolymph fills the cochlear duct while perilymph fills the scala vestibuli and scala tympani.

The ear captures vibrations and transmits resulting neural impulses to the brain for interpretation as sounds.

External Ear

The **pinna,** or ear flap, is skin with hair on the surface and underlying connective tissue. Hyaline or elastic cartilage forms the central core, and attached skeletal muscle can be contracted to move the pinna.

The **external auditory meatus,** or ear canal, is lined with skin containing fine hair, sebaceous glands and ceruminous glands. **Ceruminous glands** are modified apocrine sweat glands. Cerumen, a waxy substance from the glands, includes sebum, sloughed cells and other ceruminous gland secretions. The auditory meatus ends at the tympanic membrane.

Middle Ear

The **tympanic membrane,** or ear drum, separates the auditory meatus from the middle ear cavity. The membrane is composed of two layers of simple squamous epithelium with fine connective tissue between the epithelia.

The **tympanic cavity** is lined by simple squamous or cuboidal epithelium which covers the auditory ossicles and their muscles. **Auditory ossicles** are small bones which conduct vibrations across the middle ear cavity to the inner ear.

Lined by ciliated pseudostratified epithelium, the auditory tube (eustachian tube) connects the middle ear cavity with the pharynx

Inner Ear

The inner ear has both **osseous** and **membranous labyrinths.** The osseous labyrinth is a space within the temporal bone which contains the membranous labyrinth including the vestibular and auditory appartuses.

The **vestibular apparatus** functions in balance and proprioception. Three **semicircular canals** in the osseous labyrinth are oriented at right angles to each other. The **vestibule,** another small space in the osseous labyrinth, lies between the semicircular canals and the cochlea. **Semicircular ducts** are membranous, epithelial-lined tubules within the semicircular canals. Each duct dilates to form an **ampula** at one end. Within each ampula, sensory hair cells covered by a gelatinous cupula form the **crista ampullaris** which senses acceleration and deceleration.

The sensory cells are characterized by multiple stereocilia and a single, long kinocilium. The **utricle** and **saccule** are two membranous depressions within the vestibule. Receptor organs within these structures are the **macula utriculi** and **macula sacculi** respectively. Hair cells of the maculae and an overlying gelatinous mass with calcium carbonate crystals form the **statoconial membrane.** When the head moves, the hair cells are triggered, sending impulses along the vestibular branch of the vestibulocochlear nerve to the brain where spatial positioning is interpreted.

The **auditory apparatus** includes the **cochlea,** a spiral-shaped bony tube, and the membranous **cochlear duct** within. The cochlear duct partitions the cochlear cavity into the upper **scala vestibuli** and the lower **scala tympani.** Beginning at the vestibular window (oval window), the scala vestibuli spirals to the top of the cochlea where it bends and returns as the scala tympani which ends at the cochlear window (round window). The **vestibular membrane** separates the cochlear duct from the scala vestibuli, while the **basilar membrane** partitions the duct from the scala tympani. **Endolymph,** a clear fluid formed by the **stria vascularis,** fills the cochlear duct. **Perilymph,** derived from cerebrospinal fluid, is found in the spaces of the bony labyrinth including the scala vestibuli and scala tympani.

Within the cochlear duct, sensory and supporting cells along with the **tectorial membrane** form the **spiral organ** (organ of Corti). Axons innervating the sensory cells in the spiral organ converge and pass to the **spiral ganglion** in the center of the cochlear spiral. The cochlear branch of the vestibulocochlear nerve exits the ganglion and continues to the brain.

Auditory Mechanisms

Vibrations deflect the tympanic membrane and are transferred to the auditory ossicles of the middle ear. The ossicles then transmit the vibrations through the vestibular window into the perilymph of the cochlea. High frequency vibrations remain at the base of the cochlea while low frequency vibrations travel to the top of the spiral.   The vibrations are transferred from the perilymph to the endolymph of the cochlear duct. The basilar membrane vibrates and sensory cells deform beneath the tectorial membrane. Deformation of the sensory cells creates neural impulses which travel along the cochlear nerve to the brain for interpretation as sounds.

Questions

1. **Which of the following organelles is involved in steroid production and cell detoxification?**

   (A) agranular endoplasmic reticulum
   (B) granular andoplasmic reticulum
   (C) mitochondria
   (D) Golgi complex
   (E) ribosomes

2. **Which of the following structures are motile?**

   (A) microvilli
   (B) cilia
   (C) sterocilia
   (D) kinocilia

3. **DNA replication occurs during**

   (A Gap 1 of interphase.
   (B) S phase of interphase.
   (C) Gap 2 of interphase.
   (D) prophase of mitosis.
   (E) metaphase of mitosis.

4. **Which of the following proteins initiates the cell cycle?**

   (A) caspases
   (B) ribonucleases
   (C) cyclins
   (D) clathrin
   (E) coatomer

5. **G-protein**

   (A) mediates activity of another membrane-bound protein.
   (B) is associated with gap phases of cell division.
   (C) is found in the Golgi complex.
   (D) controls molecular transport through gap junctions.
   (E) is located in the synaptic gap between neurons.

6. **When a cell produces a signal that binds back to the producing cell, the process is called**

   (A) paracrine signaling.
   (B) endocrine signaling.
   (C) autocrine signaling.
   (D) synaptic signaling.

7. **Mesothelium is**

   (A) simple squamous epithelium that lines structures of the cardiovascular system.
   (B) simple squamous epithelium that lines body cavities.
   (C) simple cuboidal epithelium.
   (D) simple columnar epithelium.
   (E) embryonic connective tissue.

8. **Which of the following is NOT a component of the basement membrane complex?**

   (A) laminin
   (B) type IV collagen
   (C) proteoglycans
   (D) glycoproteins
   (E) keratin

9. **Endocrine glands**

   (A) have striated ducts.
   (B) include the salivary glands.
   (C) are avascular.
   (D) lack a duct system to excrete their product.
   (E) All of the above are correct.

10. **A portion of the secretory epithelial cell is lost with the product of the gland in**

    (A) merocrine secretion.
    (B) apocrine secretion.
    (C) holocrine secretion.

11. **Plasma cells**

    (A) are phagocytic.
    (B) are highly differentiated B lymphocytes.
    (C) produce proteins of blood plasma.
    (D) regulate blood vessel diameter.
    (E) develop from the fibroblast.

12. **Reticular fibers of connective tissue**

    (A) are collagen type IV.
    (B) are coated with fibronectin.
    (C) are produced by mesenchymal cells.
    (D) contain contractile filaments.
    (E) bind silver stains.

13. **Chondrocytes**

(A) reside in lacunae.
(B) synthesize collagen.
(C) can form isogenous groups.
(D) receive nutrients by diffusion through the matrix.
(E) All of the above are correct.

14. **Type I collagen is found in**

(A) hyaline cartilage.
(B) elastic cartilage.
(C) fibrocartilage.

15. **Which of the following is NOT present in spongy bone?**

(A) lacunae
(B) canaliculi
(C) lamellae
(D) osteons
(E) osteocytes

16. **The osteoclast**

(A) has a single nucleus.
(B) is multinucleated.
(C) forms bone matrix.
(D) creates a basic microenvironment for the removal of bone matrix.
(E) is derived from the fibroblast cell line.

17. **Cardiac muscle is characterized by**

(A) striated fibers, a single central nucleus and intercalated discs between cells.
(B) striated fibers, multiple peripheral nuclei, and intercalated discs between cells.
(C) non-striated fibers, a single central nucleus, and intercalated discs between cells.
(D) non-striated fibers, multiple peripheral nuclei, and intercalated discs between cells.
(E) None of the above are correct.

18. **Actin and myosin in skeletal muscle is known as**

(A) myofibrils.
(B) myofilaments.
(C) muscle fibers.
(D) microtubules.
(E) T-tubules.

19. **Axons in the central nervous system are myelinated by**

(A) neurolemmocytes.
(B) astrocytes.
(C) microglial cells.
(D) oligodendrocytes.
(E) ependymal cells.

20. **Multipolar neurons**

(A) have multiple axons.
(B) have multiple dendrites.
(C) synthesize more than one type of neurotransmitter.
(D) are multinucleated.
(E) None of the above are correct.

21. **The tunica media of blood vessels is comprised of**

(A) endothelium and underlying connective tissue.
(B) hyaline cartilage.
(C) dense irregular connective tissue.
(D) smooth muscle and connective tissue.
(E) fenestrated cells with an incomplete basal lamina.

22. **Which of the following is NOT true about sinusoids?**

(A) Sinusoids have large gaps between endothelial cells.
(B) Pores are present in the endothelial cells.
(C) An elastic membrane is present in the tunica intima.
(D) Phagocytic cells often span the lumen of a sinusoid.
(E) Sinusoids are found in bone marrow.

23. **Epicardium**

(A) is also known as parietal serous pericardium.
(B) lines the internal surface of the heart.
(C) contains cardiac conduction fibers.
(D) is anchored to the surface of the heart by the chordae tendianae.
(E) is comprised of mesothelial cells and connective tissue.

24. **Cardiac conduction fibers**

(A) have myofilaments and myofibrils in their cytoplasm.
(B) contract when stimulated by a neural impulse.
(C) conduct blood through the myocardium.
(D) anchor to cardiac valves.
(E) form pectinate muscles.

25. **Neutrophils have which of the following characteristics?**

(A) largest peripheral blood leukocyte
(B) high nuclear:cytoplasmic ratio
(C) most common granulocyte in dog and cat blood
(D) can differentiate into a plasma cell
(E) typically found in nodular-associated epithelium

26. **The erythrocyte**

(A) has a central nucleus in the dog.
(B) measures 4-7 micrometers in diameter.
(C) has cytoplasmic granules which are basophilic.
(D) has a dense tubular system for calcium transport.
(E) can be identified by the presence of Barr bodies.

27. **Structural features of a maturing blood cell can be used to stage the maturation process. A promyelocyte can be identified by**

(A) the secondary cytoplasmic granules.
(B) a prominent nucleolus.
(C) the condensation of polyribosomes when stained with a vital stain.
(D) primary granules.
(E) a large polyploid nucleus.

28. **Which of the following forms the supporting structure of bone marrow?**

(A) collagen fiber framework
(B) macrophages which phagocytize spent cells
(C) reticular cells
(D) epithelial reticular cells
(E) megakaryocytes

29. **In the hypophysis cerebri, adrenocorticotrophic hormone is produced by**

(A) pituicytes.
(B) somatotropes.
(C) lactotropes.
(D) gonadotropes.
(E) corticotropes.

30. **The hypophysial portal system**

(A) transports hormones to the neurohypophysis.
(B) consists of axons from the supraoptic and paraventricular nuclei.
(C) connects the hypophyis cerebri to the liver.
(D) transports hypothalamic secretions to the cells in the pars distalis.
(E) connects the pars distalis to the neurohypophysis.

31. **In the horse, principal cells and oxyphil cells are found in the**

(A) thyroid gland.
(B) parathyroid gland.
(C) suprarenal gland.
(D) neurohypophysis.
(E) epiphysis cerebri.

32. **Thyroid follicular lining cells**

(A) form a stratified epithelium which lines the follicles.
(B) secrete colloid across the basal cell membrane into surrounding capillaries.
(C) are fenestrated.
(D) form gap junctions with parafollicular cells.
(E) take up circulating iodide from the blood.

33. **The zona fasiculata**

(A) is located in the suprarenal medulla.
(B) contains cells which secrete insulin.
(C) has cells with large numbers of cytoplasmic lipid droplets.
(D) produces epinephrine and norepinephrine.
(E) has mineralized bodies known as corpora aranacea.

34. **Medullary endocrine cells of the suprarenal medulla**

(A) are directly innervated by preganglionic sympathetic nerve fibers.
(B) are stimulated by ACTH from the hypophysis.
(C) produce mineralocorticoids.
(D) produce glucocorticoids.
(E) do not stain with the chromaffin technique.

35. **Which of the following cells in the pancreas produces insulin?**

(A) A cell
(B) B cell
(C) D cell
(D) pancreatic polypeptide cell
(E) All of the above cells produce insulin.

36. **Centroacinar cells**

(A) produce zymogen granules.
(B) contract to help expel acinar contents.
(C) are extensions of the intercalated duct epithelium into the lumen of the acinus.
(D) regulate gastrointestinal activity.
(E) produce mucus.

37. **Which of the following components is NOT present in the blood-thymic barrier?**

(A) epithelial reticular cell
(B) endothelial cell
(C) endothelial cell basement membrane
(D) macrophage
(E) perivascular connective tissue

38. **Thymic corpuscles are located in the**

(A) cortex of the thymus.
(B) medulla of the thymus.

39. **The predominant cell of the germinal center of an active lymphatic nodule is the**

(A) B lymphocyte.
(B) T lymphocyte.

40. **High endothelial vessels**

(A) have a stratified epithelial lining.
(B) transport and filter lymph.
(C) allow lymphocytes to leave the blood and enter the lymph node.
(D) connect to the subcapsular sinus.
(E) have stellate reticular cells which span the lumen.

41. **The marginal zone of the spleen is located**

(A) between the capsule and the subcapsular sinus.
(B) immediately surrounding the nodular artery.
(C) between the white pulp and the periarteriolar lymphatic sheath (PALS).
(D) between the red pulp and the white pulp.
(E) in the medullary region near efferent lymphatics.

42. **The periarteriolar lymphatic sheath (PALS) of the spleen**

(A) is a B cell zone.
(B) is located within the germinal center of a splenic nodule.
(C) surrounds an artery of the white pulp.
(D) surrounds a terminal capillary.
(E) contains plasma cells as the major cell type.

43. Which of the following cells are present in epithelium located over gut-associated lymphatic nodules?

(A) goblet cells
(B) plasma cells
(C) microfold cells
(D) principal cells
(E) centroacinar cells

44. Crypts are deep invaginations of the surface epithelium in the

(A) palatine tonsil.
(B) pharyngeal tonsil.
(C) lingual tonsil.
(D) ileal aggregated lymphatic nodules.
(E) bronchiolar-associated lymphatic tissue.

45. In tubular organs, smooth muscle is present in the

(A) mucosal epithelium.
(B) lamina muscularis.
(C) tunica muscularis.
(D) lamina muscularis and tunica muscularis.
(E) All of the above are correct.

46. Which of the following layers is found on the surface of organs adjacent to the peritoneal cavity?

(A) mucosal epithelium
(B) lamina muscularis
(C) lamina propria
(D) tunica adventitia
(E) tunica serosa

47. The first level where oxygen can cross into blood circulation occurs at the

(A) respiratory epithelium in the nasal cavity.
(B) larynx.
(C) trachea.
(D) bronchus.
(E) bronchiole with alveoli.

48. Olfactory epithelium does NOT have

(A) sustentacular cells.
(B) bipolar neurons.
(C) goblet cells.
(D) basal cells.

49. The proximal tubules of the kidney are lined by

(A) simple cuboidal epithelium with tight intercellular junctions.
(B) simple cuboidal epithelium with leaky intercellular junctions.
(C) simple squamous epithelium.
(D) simple columnar epithelium with goblet cells.
(E) transitional epithelium.

50. Podocytes

(A) are part of the juxtaglomerular apparatus.
(B) contact the macula densa.
(C) form the visceral layer of the glomerular capsule.
(D) have cilia on their surface.
(E) produce bicarbonate in the urine.

51. The urethra can be differentiated from the ureter by the presence of

(A) transitional epithelium lining the lumen.
(B) smooth muscle in the tunica muscularis.
(C) cavernous vascular spaces in the propria-submucosa.
(D) prominent ganglia between muscle layers.
(E) a tunica adventitia as the outer layer.

52. Which species has goblet cells and mucous glands in the ureter?

(A) canine
(B) feline
(C) bovine
(D) equine
(E) porcine

53. Interstitial cells

(A) produce testosterone.
(B) are located in the wall of the seminiferous tubules.
(C) are a component of the blood-testes barrier.
(D) support spermatogenic cells.
(E) line the rete testis.

54. The prostate is lined by

(A) simple cuboidal epithelium.
(B) stratified columnar epithelium.
(C) simple columnar epithelium.
(D) pseudostratified epithelium.
(E) mucous epithelium.

55. In the ovary, androgens are produced by the

(A) zona pellucida.
(B) corona radiata.
(C) theca interna.
(D) theca externa.
(E) tunica albuginea.

56. Stratified squamous epithelium lines the

(A) pre-ovulatory atretic follicle.
(B) uterine tube.
(C) uterus.
(D) cervix.
(E) vagina.

57. All three maternal layers are intact in what type of placenta?

(A) epitheliochorial
(B) synepitheliochorial
(C) endotheliochorial
(D) hemochorial
(E) deciduate

58. Endometrial cups

(A) are found along the edge of the canine placenta.
(B) form from allantoic endoderm.
(C) produce horse chorionic gonadotropin.
(D) form opposite uterine glands.
(E) appear at 150 days gestation.

59. Dentine is produced by

(A) enameloblasts.
(B) odontoblasts.
(C) cementoblasts.
(D) fibroblasts.
(E) pulp cavity cells.

60. Serous salivary glands can be differentiated from exocrine pancreas by the presence of

(A) goblet cells.
(B) zymogen granules.
(C) striated ducts.
(D) reticular fibers in the connective tissue stroma.
(E) stratified columnar epithelium lining ducts.

61. Striated muscle is found in the tunica muscularis throughout the length of the esophagus in the

(A) horse.
(B) pig.
(C) dog.
(D) cat.
(E) All of the above are correct.

62. Hydrochloric acid in the stomach is produced by

(A) epithelial cells of the cardiac glands.
(B) the myenteric plexus.
(C) mucous neck cells.
(D) principal cells.
(E) parietal cells.

63. Goblet cells in the intestine

(A) are confined to submucosal glands.
(B) increase in number from the small intestine to the rectum.
(C) empty into lacteals.
(D) produce peptidase.
(E) present antigens to underlying GALT.

64. Circumanal glands

(A) have intercalated ducts which empty into the anal canal.
(B) produce secretions which are stored in the anal sac.
(C) are surrounded by smooth muscle of the external anal sphincter.
(D) are derived from sebaceous glands.
(E) contain mucous cells.

65. The perisinusoidal space in the liver contains

(A) plasma.
(B) stellate macrophage cells.
(C) bile.
(D) connective tissue.
(E) pericytes.

66. The central vein forms the central structure of the

(A) liver lobe.
(B) liver acinus.
(C) portal lobule.
(D) hepatic lobule.
(E) biliary system.

67. Melanocytes

(A) are clear cells.
(B) are brown due to melanin pigment.
(C) renew during catagen.
(D) are phagocytized by intraepidermal macrophages.
(E) are most numerous in the stratum granulosum.

68. The principal sweat gland of animals is

(A) merocrine.
(B) apocrine.
(C) holocrine.
(D) sebaceous.
(E) mucous.

69. The stratum tectorium of the equine hoof is produced by the

(A) stratum lamellatum.
(B) coronary corium.
(C) coronary epidermis.
(D) perioplic corium.
(E) perioplic epidermis.

70. The hoof wall grows

(A) in a ring-like fashion from the stratum medium.
(B) from cells in the white line.
(C) from cells in the coronary corium.
(D) from cells in the laminar corium.
(E) as horn is added at the coronary epidermis.

71. The formation of a secondary center of ossification is initiated by

(A) woven bone.
(B) the physis.
(C) a vascular bud in the cartilage canals.
(D) the primary center of ossification.
(E) the perichondrium.

72. The advancing edge of metaphyseal blood vessels is found in which zone of the physis?

(A) reserve
(B) proliferating
(C) hypertrophying
(D) resorbing
(E) ossification

73. The calcified layer of articular cartilage is located in the

(A) superficial zone.
(B) middle zone.
(C) deep zone.

74. Which of the following structures is NOT fibrocartilage?

(A) menisci
(B) articular cartilage
(C) insertion of ligaments into bone
(D) symphysis
(E) endotendineum

75. The tapetum lucidum is located in the

(A) retina.
(B) choroid.
(C) sclera.
(D) iris.
(E) lens.

76. Aqueous humor

(A) is produced by the lens.
(B) flows from the ciliary body through the iris to the iridial angle.
(C) is produced by zonular fibers.
(D) originates from the stratum avasculorum.
(E) is produced by the posterior epithelium of the cornea.

77. Which of the following structures is NOT involved in hearing?

(A) semicircular canals
(B) scala vestibuli
(C) stria vascularis
(D) perilymph
(E) tectorial membrane

78. Ceruminous glands are

(A) mucous glands.
(B) sebaceous glands.
(C) modified sweat glands.
(D) located in the auditory tube.
(E) attached to the inner surface of the tympanic membrane.

Answers

1. **A**	31. **B**	61. **C**
2. **B**	32. **E**	62. **E**
3. **B**	33. **C**	63. **B**
4. **C**	34. **A**	64. **D**
5. **A**	35. **B**	65. **A**
6. **C**	36. **C**	66. **D**
7. **B**	37. **D**	67. **A**
8. **E**	38. **B**	68. **B**
9. **D**	39. **A**	69. **E**
10. **B**	40. **C**	70. **E**
11. **B**	41. **D**	71. **C**
12. **E**	42. **C**	72. **D**
13. **E**	43. **C**	73. **C**
14. **C**	44. **A**	74. **E**
15. **D**	45. **D**	75. **B**
16. **B**	46. **E**	76. **B**
17. **A**	47. **E**	77. **A**
18. **B**	48. **C**	78. **C**
19. **D**	49. **B**	
20. **B**	50. **C**	
21. **D**	51. **C**	
22. **C**	52. **D**	
23. **E**	53. **A**	
24. **A**	54. **D**	
25. **C**	55. **C**	
26. **B**	56. **E**	
27. **D**	57. **A**	
28. **C**	58. **C**	
29. **E**	59. **B**	
30. **D**	60. **C**	

References

Alberts B, et al. *Molecular Biology of the Cell.* New York: Garland, 1994.

American Association of Equine Practitioners. *Official Guide for Determining the Age of the Horse.* AAEP monograph, 1988.

Banks WJ. *Applied Veterinary Histology.* St. Louis: Mosby Year Book, 1993.

Baserga R. The cell cycle. New Eng J Med 304(8): 453-459, 1981.

Boyett MR, et al. The sinoatrial node, a heterogeneous pacemaker structure. Cardiovasc Res 47:658-687, 2000.

Dellmann H-D, Eurell J (eds). *Textbook of Veterinary Histology.* Baltimore: Lippincott, Williams and Wilkins, 1998.

Evans HE, Christensen GC. *Miller's Anatomy of the Dog.* Philadelphia: WB Saunders, 1979.

Fawcett DW, Jensh RP. *Bloom & Fawcett: Concise Histology.* New York: Chapman and Hall, 1997.

Gartner LP, Hiatt JL. *Color Textbook of Histology.* Philadelphia: WB Saunders, 2001.

Ghohestani R, et al. Molecular organization of the cutaneous basement membrane zone. Clin Dermatol 19:551-562, 2001.

James TN, et al. Anatomy of the heart. In: Hurst JW. *The Heart, Arteries and Veins.* New York: McGraw-Hill, 1982.

Junqueira LC, Carneiro J. *Basic Histology.* New York: Lange, 2003.

Kelly DE, et al. *Bailey's Textbook of Microscopic Anatomy.* Baltimore: Williams and Wilkins, 1984.

Kerr JB. *Atlas of Functional Histology.* St. Louis: Mosby, 1999.

Keverne EB. The vomeronasal organ. Science 286:716-720, 1999.

Mankin HJ, et al. Form and function of articular cartilage. In: Simon SR (ed). *Orthopedic Basic Science.* Park Ridge: American Academy of Orthopaedic Surgeons, 1994.

Nickel T, et al. *The Viscera of Domestic Mammals.* New York: Springer-Verlag, 1973.

Parslow TG, et al. *Medical Immunology.* New York: McGraw-Hill, 2001.

Pollitt CC. *Color Atlas of the Horse's Foot.* Baltimore: Mosby-Wolfe, 1995.

Stump JE. Anatomy of the normal equine foot, including microscopic features of the laminar region. JAVMA 151(12): 1588-1598, 1967.

Trautmann A, Fiebiger J. *Fundamentals of the Histology of Domestic Animals.* Ithaca: Comstock, 1957.

Winoto A. Genes involved in T-cell receptor-mediated apoptosis of thymocytes and T-cell hybridomas. Semin Immunol 9(1):51-8, 1997.

Woo S, et al. Ligament, tendon, and joint capsule insertions to bone. In: Woo SL-Y, Buckwalter JA (eds). *Injury and Repair of the Musculoskeletal Soft Tissues.* Park Ridge: American Academy of Orthopaedic Surgeons, 1988.

Index

mucosal, 47
pigmented, 77
posterior surface of eye, 77
pseudostratified, 8-9
respiratory, 49
simple, 8-9
squamous, 9, 49, 61
stratified columnar, 8-9
stratified cuboidal, 8-9
transitional, 8-9
Epithielioid cells, 21
Epsilon cells, 31
Equine hoof, 70-71
Ergot, 69
Erosion cavity, 17
Erythrocytes, 26-27
maturation of, 29
Erythrocytic cell series, 29
Erythropoietin, 29
Esophagus, 62-63
Estrogen
follicular cell production of, 57
suprarenal production of, 35
Euchromatin, 3
formation of, 5
Exocrine ducts, 11, 37
Exocrine glands, 11
Exocrine secretory units, 37
Extraembryonic membranes, 59
Eye
compartments of, 77
fibrous tunic of, 77
structures of, 76, 77
vascular layer of, 77
vascular tunic of, 77
Eyelid, 77

F cell, 37
Fabricus, bursa of, 45
Fenestrated capillaries, 23
in suprarenal gland, 35
Fetus, 59
Fibrinogen, 27
Fibroblast synovial cells, 75
Fibroblasts, 13
Fibrocartilage, 15, 75
Fibrocytes, 13
Fibronectin, 13
Fibrous pericardium, 25
Fibrous tunic, 77
Filiform papillae, 61
Filtration slit, renal, 51
Flagella, 3
Foliate folds, 61
Follicle stimulating hormone, 31
Follicular dendritic cells, 41
Follicular development, 57
Follicular lining cells, 33

Fungiform papillae, 61

G cell, 37
G-protein-linked receptor, 7
Gallbladder, 66-67
Gamma-globulins, 27
Ganglia, 21
Ganglia gliocytes, 21
Ganglion cells, 35
of eye, 77
Gap 1 phase, 5
Gap 2 phase, 5
Gap junction, 9
cell signaling and, 7
Gas exchange, across blood-air barrier, 49
Gastric folds, 63
Gastric glands, 63
Gastric inhibitory protein, 37
Gastric pits, 63
Gastrin, 37
Germinal center, 41
Gestation, 59
Gingival sulcus, 61
Glands, 10
anal, 65
of anal sac, 65
ceruminous, 79
classification of, 11
intestinal, 65
olfactory, 49
secretions of, 11
of skin, 69
of stomach, 63
suprarenal, 34–35
Glans penis, 55
Glassy membrane, 69
Gliocytes, radial, 77
Glomerular arterioles, 51
Glomerular capsule, 51
Glomerulus, 51
Glucagon, 37
Glucocorticoids, 35
Glycocalyx, 3
Glycogen
breakdown of, 37
cellular, 3
Glycogenolysis, 37
Glycosaminoglycans (GAGs), 13, 15
Goblet cells, 11
intestinal, 65
Golgi apparatus, 37
Golgi complex, 3
Gonadotropes, 31
Granular cells
acidophilic, 65
in tunica media, 51
Granulocytes, 27
immature, 29

S phase, 5
Saccule, 79
Salivary glands, 11, 60-61
  cells of, 61
Sarcolemma, 19
Sarcoplasm, 19
Sarcoplasmic reticulum, 19
Satellite cells, 21
Scala tympani, 79
Scala vestibuli, 79
Schwann cell, 21
Sclera, 77
Scrotum, 54-55
Sebaceous glands, 69
Secretion, modes of, 11
Secretory cells, 11
Secretory granules, 3
Secretory units, exocrine, 11
Semicircular canals, 79
Semicircular ducts, 79
Seminal vesicle, 55
Seminiferous tubules
  convoluted, 55
  straight, 55
Sensory gustatory cells, 61
Sensory hairs, 69
Seromucous secretion, 11
Serotonin, 31
Serous cells, salivary, 61
Serous demilune, 11
Serous secretion, 11
Sertoli cells, 55
Serum, 27
Sharpey's fiber, 75
Signaling cell, 7
Sinoatrial node, 25
Sinuses
  for blood transport, 23
  of lymph nodes, 41
  in lymph transport, 23
  medullary, 41
  splenic, 43
Sinusoidal endothelial cells, 67
Sinusoids, 23
Skeletal muscle, 18, 19
  A band of, 19
  I band fibers of, 19
  of tongue, 61
Skin
  glands associated with, 69
  layers of, 68-69
Slit diaphragm, 51
Sodium ions, 21
Soft palate, 61
Somatotropes, 31
Somatotropin, 31
Spectrin, 27
Spermatic cord, 55
Spermatid, 55

Spermatocytes
  primary, 55
  secondary, 55
Spermatogenic cells, 55
Spermatogonium, 55
Spermatozoon, 55
Sphincter muscle, ocular, 77
Spiral ganglion, 79
Spiral organ, 79
Spleen
  blood filtration mechanisms in, 43
  blood supply to, 43
  capsule of, 43
  marginal zone of, 43
  red pulp of, 43
  structures of, 42
  white pulp of, 43
Splenic cords, 43
Squamous cells, epidermal, 69
Squamous epithelium
  of nose, 49
  oral, 61
  simple, 9
  stratified, 9
Statoconial membrane, 79
Stellate macrophage cells, 67
Stem cells
  committed, 29
  hematopoietic, 12
  uncommitted hemocytopoietic, 29
Stereocilia, 3
Stomach, 62–63
  monogastric, 63
Stratum avasculorum, 77
Stratum basale, 69
Stratum compactum, 63
Stratum corneum, 69
Stratum granulosum, 57, 69
Stratum lamellatum, 71
Stratum lucidum, 69
Stratum medium, hoof, 71
Stratum spinosum, 69
Stratum tectorium, 71
Stria vascularis, 79
Striated duct, salivary, 61
Stroma, 11, 21
  of adenohypophysis, 31
  of eye, 77
Subendothelium, 23
Submucosal glands
  intestinal, 65
  of male urethra, 55
Submucosal plexus, stomach, 63
Substantia propria, 77
Suprachoroid, 77
Suprarenal gland
  blood supply to, 35
  cortex of, 35
  structures of, 34-35